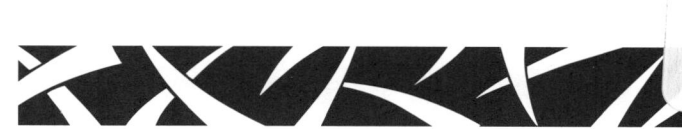

Parent Articles About NDT

Edited by Rhoda P. Erhardt, M.S., OTR, FAOTA

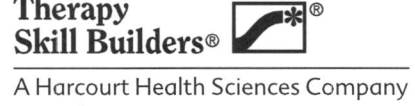

A Harcourt Health Sciences Company

Reproducing Pages From This Book

As described below, some of the pages in this book may be reproduced for instructional use (not for resale). To protect your book, make a photocopy of each reproducible page. Then use that copy as a master for photocopying.

Copyright © 1999 by

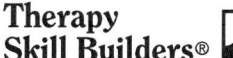 

A Harcourt Health Sciences Company

All rights reserved. No part of this publication may be reproduced or transmitted in any form or by any means, electronic or mechanical, including photocopy, recording, or any information storage and retrieval system, without permission in writing from the publisher.

Permission is hereby granted to reproduce the articles in this publication in complete pages, with the copyright notice, for instructional use and not for resale.

The *Learning Curve Design* and *Therapy Skill Builders* are registered trademarks of The Psychological Corporation.

Some material in this work previously appeared in *Pediatric Massage for the Child with Special Needs*, copyright © 1991 by Kathy Fleming Drehobl and Mary Gengler Fuhr, published by Therapy Skill Builders, a division of The Psychological Corporation, and *Spatial, Temporal, and Physical Analysis of Motor Control: A Comprehensive Guide to Reflexes and Reactions*, copyright © 1997 by Diane Berg McCormack and Kathy Riske Perrin, published by Therapy Skill Builders, a division of The Psychological Corporation.

Illustrations for Articles 2.3, 3.1, 3.2, 3.3, 3.6, 4.1, 4.2, 4.11, 5.3, 5.5, 5.7, and 6.4 drawn under contract by Irene Maag.

Illustrations 4a and 4b in Article 3.3 and illustration 1 in Article 4.2 drawn under contract by Exhibit A Productions.

0761641009

1 2 3 4 5 6 7 8 9 10 11 12 A B C D E

Printed in the United States of America

Visit our website at www.tpcweb.com. To contact Therapy Skill Builders, call 1-800-228-0752.

Contents

How to Use This Book 1

Section 1: Neuro-Developmental Treatment

    1.1   In the Beginning: Berta and Karel Bobath
           (Jay Schleichkorn, Ph.D., PT) 7

    1.2   Philosophy, Theory, and Principles:
           The What, Why, and How of NDT (Judith Bierman, PT) 11

Section 2: Social/Emotional Aspects

    2.1   The Emotional Aspects of Having a Child With Disabilities
           (Suzanne M. Davis, RPT) 15

    2.2   Coping: Movement Made Meaningful
           (G. Gordon Williamson, Ph.D., OTR) 19

    2.3   The Autonomic Nervous System: Support for Life
           (Cynthia Lewis, Ph.D., PT) 23

Section 3: Posture and Positioning

    3.1   Postural Control: Stability for Function (Barbara Cupps, PT) ... 29

    3.2   Quality of Movement: The Importance of Postural Control for
           Functional Activity (Linda King-Thomas, M.H.S., OTR/L) 33

    3.3   Is W-Sitting a Problem? Managing the Modeling of Bone
           and Joint Geometry (Beverly Cusick, M.S., PT) 37

    3.4   Orthotics/Orthoses/Braces/Splints:
           What Could They Mean for Your Child? (Allison Whiteside, PT) .. 45

    3.5   These Arms Are Meant for Reaching:
           Upper-Extremity Casting for Functional Alignment
           (Audrey Yasukawa, M.O.T., OTR/L) 49

    3.6   How Can I Get That Arm Straight? The Quest for
           Elbow Extension (Diane Berg McCormack, M.S., OTR) 53

Section 4: Movement and Touch

    4.1   Learning to Move (Gloria Frolek Clark, M.S., OTR/L, FAOTA) .. 59

    4.2   Practicing Basic Transitions: Foundations for All
           Movement Skills (Vickie Meade, M.P.H., PT) 63

    4.3   A Positive Perspective on Atypical Development:
           Understanding Why Your Child Moves This Way
           (Suzanne M. Davis, RPT) 67

    4.4   Minimizing the Problem of Learned Helplessness:
           What Can Parents Do to Help? (Kristen Birkmeier, M.S., PT) ... 69

    4.5   The Unique Physical Challenges of Children With Hypertonia
           (Marcia Stamer, PT) 71

    4.6   The Unique Physical Challenges of Children With Hypotonia
           (Marcia Stamer, PT) 73

4.7	The Unique Physical Challenges of Children With Athetosis (Marcia Stamer, PT)	75
4.8	The Unique Physical Challenges of Children With Ataxia (Marcia Stamer, PT)	77
4.9	Making Movement Easier Through Touch (Regi Boehme, OTR)	79
4.10	Touching Is Fun! Helping Children Learn to Use Their Hands (Lezlie Adler, M.A., OTR, FMOT)	81
4.11	Handling With Care or Handling Carefully: Sensory Problems in Infants With Cerebral Palsy (Mary Hallway, OTR)	85

Section 5: Personal Care

5.1	Too Young, Too Soon: Sucking and Swallowing in the Preterm Infant (Robin González, SLP)	95
5.2	Help Me Learn to Eat: Sensory Experiences to Facilitate Feeding Skills (Merry M. Meek, M.S., CCC-Sp)	99
5.3	Sit Up at the Dinner Table! Feeding Positioning Tips for Parents (Gay Lloyd Pinder, Ph.D., CCC-SLP)	101
5.4	Tube-Feeding Decisions: The What, When, Why, and How (Marybeth Trapani-Hanasewych, M.S., CCC-SLP)	105
5.5	Drooling: Ways to Manage a Difficult Problem (Janet H. Allaire, M.A., CCC-SLP)	107
5.6	Caring Strokes for Little Folks: Therapeutic Pediatric Massage (Kathy Fleming Drehobl, B.S., OTR/L, and Mary Gengler Fuhr, B.S., OTR/L)	111
5.7	Leaning and Lifting: Practical Use of Weight Shifts for Adolescents and Adults (Laura Vogtle, Ph.D., OTR/L)	115

Section 6: Play and Recreation

6.1	Play or Therapy? Make Time for Both! (Anita Bundy, Sc.D., OTR, FAOTA)	121
6.2	Why Children Love to Play: The Importance of Intrinsic Motivation (Erna I. Blanche, Ph.D., OTR)	123
6.3	Vision: Must It Stand Alone? (Rhoda P. Erhardt, M.S., OTR, FAOTA)	125
6.4	Buoyancy-Assisted Function Through Therapeutic Aquatics (Jane Styer-Acevedo, PT)	129
6.5	Hippotherapy: Treatment With the Help of the Horse (Linda Kliebhan, PT)	133
6.6	Getting Pumped Up for Therapy During the Teen Years: Working Through the Stress of Adolescence (Madonna Nash, OTR)	135

Section 7: Communication and School Activities

7.1	To Speak Is the Greatest Gift: Facilitating Oral-Motor Coordination for Speech Production (Merry M. Meek, M.S., CCC-Sp)	141
7.2	Reading: Opening Communication Interactions (Deborah Minteer, M.S., CCC-SLP)	143

        7.3   Layering: An Art of Therapy
                (Judy Michels Jelm, M.S., CCC-SLP) 145
        7.4   Can I Sign on the Dotted Line?? (Regi Boehme, OTR) 147

Section 8: Roles
        8.1   Parents Have Learning Styles Too! How to Help Your
                Therapist Help You Help Your Child
                (Marsha Dunn Klein, M.Ed., OTR/L) 151
        8.2   Parents and Therapists as Collaborators in Therapy Programs
                (Kristen Birkmeier, M.S., PT) 155
        8.3   Divide Up the Tasks, Not the Body Parts
                (Marybeth Trapani-Hanasewych, M.S., CCC-SLP) 157
        8.4   Team Goals and Roles: How Parents Can Assure
                Continuity of Care (Diane Berg McCormack, M.S., OTR) 159
        8.5   What Does My Child Need and How Can I Help?
                Application and Philosophy of NDT According to the Bobaths
                (Joan Mohr, PT) 163

References for Parents 165

Contributing Authors

Article Number

Lezlie Adler, M.A., OTR, FMOT	4.10
Janet H. Allaire, M.A., CCC-SLP	5.5
Judith Bierman, PT	1.2
Kristen Birkmeier, M.S., PT	4.4, 8.2
Erna I. Blanche, Ph.D., OTR	6.2
Regi Boehme, OTR	4.9, 7.4
Anita Bundy, Sc.D., OTR, FAOTA	6.1
Gloria Frolek Clark, M.S., OTR/L, FAOTA	4.1
Barbara Cupps, PT	3.1
Beverly Cusick, M.S., PT	3.3
Suzanne M. Davis, RPT	2.1, 4.3
Kathy Fleming Drehobl, B.S., OTR/L	5.6
Rhoda P. Erhardt, M.S., OTR, FAOTA	6.3
Mary Gengler Fuhr, B.S., OTR/L	5.6
Robin González, SLP	5.1
Mary Hallway, OTR	4.11
Judy Michels Jelm, M.S., CCC-SLP	7.3
Linda King-Thomas, M.H.S., OTR/L	3.2
Marsha Dunn Klein, M.Ed., OTR/L	8.1
Linda Kliebhan, PT	6.5
Cynthia Lewis, Ph.D., PT	2.3
Diane Berg McCormack, M.S., OTR	3.6, 8.4
Vickie Meade, M.P.H., PT	4.2
Merry M. Meek, M.S., CCC-Sp	5.2, 7.1
Deborah Minteer, M.S., CCC-SLP	7.2
Joan Mohr, PT	8.5
Madonna Nash, OTR	6.6
Gay Lloyd Pinder, Ph.D., CCC-SLP	5.3
Jay Schleichkorn, Ph.D., PT	1.1
Marcia Stamer, PT	4.5, 4.6, 4.7, 4.8
Jane Styer-Acevedo, PT	6.4
Marybeth Trapani-Hanasewych, M.S., CCC-SLP	5.4, 8.3
Laura Vogtle, Ph.D., OTR/L	5.7
Allison Whiteside, PT	3.4
G. Gordon Williamson, Ph.D., OTR	2.2
Audrey Yasukawa, M.O.T., OTR/L	3.5

About the Editor

Rhoda Priest Erhardt, M.S., OTR, FAOTA, received her bachelor of science degree in occupational therapy from the University of Illinois and her master's degree in child development and family relations from North Dakota State University. She was trained in pediatric Neuro-Developmental treatment (NDT) in London, England.

The former director of the Easter Seal Mobile Therapy Unit in Fargo, North Dakota, Mrs. Erhardt currently is in private practice in the Minneapolis/St. Paul area, providing evaluation and consultation services to a variety of health agencies, educational systems, and national corporations, as well as presenting workshops throughout the world. She has served on the editorial board of the *American Journal of Occupational Therapy* and the Board of Occupational Therapy Practice of North Dakota, and was enrolled in the American Occupational Therapy Association (AOTA) Roster of Fellows in 1983.

Mrs. Erhardt's publications include books, chapters, journal articles, assessments, and videotapes on topics such as prehension, vision, eye-hand coordination, and feeding problems in children with cerebral palsy as well as perceptual problems in children with learning disabilities. Her videotape on normal hand development received an award from the American Academy for Cerebral Palsy and Developmental Medicine.

How to Use This Book

Marsha Dunn Klein, M.Ed., OTR/L, and Rhoda P. Erhardt, M.S., OTR, FAOTA

Purpose of the Book

Parent Articles About NDT is a collection of reproducible handouts on topics related to the theories of Neuro-Developmental Treatment (NDT) taught initially by Karl and Berta Bobath. Many parents will enjoy reading the first article in the book, which introduces the Bobaths and explains how and why they became concerned about and interested in children with cerebral palsy.

These handouts have many uses:

1. New therapists can use these articles to clarify or consolidate their thinking about the application of neuro-developmental principles in treatment.

2. Advanced physical therapists, occupational therapists, and speech-language pathologists can read about the current treatment theories and approaches in the writings of colleagues.

3. The primary purpose of these articles is for all therapists to reproduce individual handouts for parents. Each article is meant to stand alone as a single handout for a family of a child with disabilities. The treating therapist should read each article carefully to be sure the information is appropriate to share with a particular parent about his or her child. It is our hope that parents of children with disabilities will find the information helpful in expanding their understanding of NDT theory and how it influences the therapy for their child. At the end of each article is the suggestion that Judith Bierman's article 1.2, "Philosophy, Theory, and Principles: The What, Why, and How of NDT," offers more clarification on that topic.

No handout can cover all possible treatment variations and principles. Sometimes the therapist will use the handout as a beginning focus of discussion, adding his or her own ideas to the printed ones. Other times, the handouts will complement the information already shared during a specific session. Therapists must decide whether a certain article is appropriate for parents whose child is just starting therapy or for those whose child has been in therapy for years.

Organization and Listing of Contents by Title

We had considerable discussion about how to arrange these articles for the reader. Do we organize the material by physical therapy, occupational therapy, or speech therapy? Do we use the old standby of leg-related articles for physical therapy, arm-related articles for occupational therapy, and mouth-related articles for speech therapy? No! Those artificial divisions were exactly what the Bobaths were trying to avoid. A basic principle of NDT treatment theory is that characteristics and functioning of one part of the body influence characteristics and functioning of other parts of the body. For example, we do not work on walking without treating the trunk and shoulders. We do not look at hand function without being very aware of the influences of the trunk and hips. And we do not focus on speech without careful understanding of the head, neck, and trunk. We must look at the whole picture before we can do a good job of treating a specific area in order to facilitate a specific function.

It is important for us to remember that NDT does not exist in isolation. Therapists use NDT with a variety of other modalities, theoretical approaches, and therapies, all providing foundations for function. Because the NDT-trained authors have kept themselves informed about current research and practice trends, they have incorporated theories and concepts such as sensory integration, motor control, and kinesiology into their work. For example, several handouts contain information about casting and splinting, which might be essential treatment components for some children to achieve alignment, which is the basis for posture.

So, we arranged the handouts using the same general umbrella of organization that all NDT-trained therapists use to look at children. We have begun by giving you important background information about the Bobaths, and why and how they came to make such an important contribution to individuals with cerebral palsy (CP). Next, we wanted to share with you the most current information about NDT theory, which is evolving constantly.

First and foremost, the Bobaths always considered the children's emotional and social needs, which influenced and were influenced by basic survival functions. NDT is all about understanding the whole body and how movement relates to all function. Therefore, the handouts next address posture and movement. There are articles about postural control, learning to move, and transitions involving upper and lower extremities.

A good understanding of movement and posture helps us appreciate the handouts about touch and handling. Touch influences the child's interactions with the environment as well as the therapist's physical interactions with the child. This information on movement and touch is central to treating children with disabilities.

The Bobaths also taught us to look beyond specific movements and therapeutic handling techniques. They taught us to focus on function. For a child, that function can include moving everywhere possible to explore everything possible, playing with all kinds of toys and performing activities of daily living such as eating, dressing, toileting, and toothbrushing. Some handouts in this book use functional activities as examples of an NDT principle. In other handouts that focus is on analysis of a specific functional task and examples of several NDT principles that relate to it.

Communication is layered on the postural tone and movement base and integrated into all activities of daily living. The child must be able to use posture and movement to control the muscle patterns needed to communicate. Positive interaction between the child and the therapist, and more importantly, between the child and the family, are key to the therapeutic process.

And finally, we have handouts that look at the roles of parents and therapists in this partnership of treatment of children. Whose job is it to do what? What can we do to adapt our goals and treatment methods throughout the children's life spans? How can therapists and parents work together to improve their quality of life?

List of Contributing Authors

Once you have familiarized yourself with the book and the authors, you will be able to locate a particular handout quickly by looking up the author name in the Contributing Authors list, which is alphabetized for quick retrieval.

The Future

These handouts only scratch the surface of information to be shared. You might read a handout and wish it had taken another focus, or you might search for a handout on a particular topic and find that it was not included. You might want to share information on an NDT-related topic that a parent has found especially useful. Perhaps you even can suggest a person who would be a good author for that or other articles, or you yourself might want to write on topics you want included. Following is a *Parent Articles About NDT* topic-suggestion form. Take time to look it over. Whenever you have a suggestion that should be included in the next NDT articles book, please write it down and send it to Therapy Skill Builders. We look forward to hearing from you.

Suggestions for a future book of NDT articles

Topic: _____

Function: _____

Author: _____

Potential-Author Address: _____

Potential-Author Phone: _____

Please return to: Acquisitions Editor
Therapy Skill Builders
555 Academic Court
San Antonio, TX 78204-2498

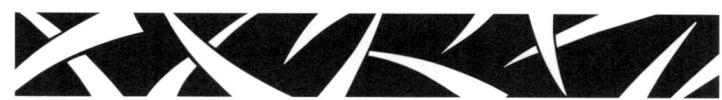

Section 1

Neuro-Developmental Treatment

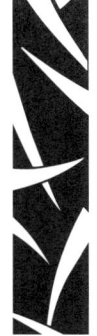

In the Beginning: Berta and Karel Bobath

Jay Schleichkorn, Ph.D., PT
Photo by Phil Weedon

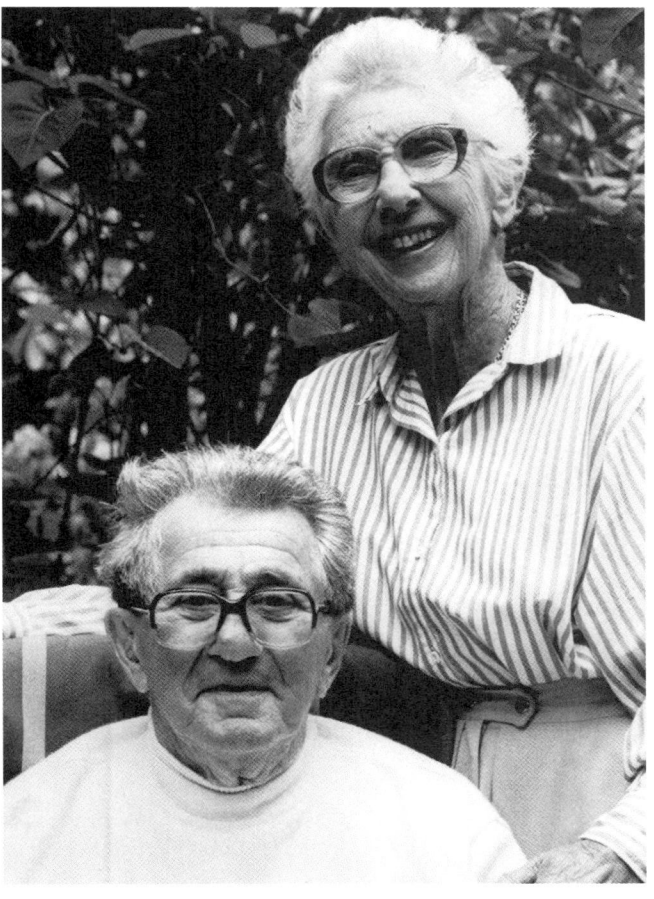

The Bobaths at home, September 1990.

How often have we heard the expression "being in the right place at the right time with the right idea?" We need only to look at the many conveniences we enjoy today because of someone's concept, initiative, or invention. Fortunately for thousands of children and adults with cerebral palsy (CP), their families, and the community, Berta and Karel Bobath spent about 80 years each on our planet and left a legacy that will not be forgotten: Neuro-Developmental Treatment (NDT).

The Bobaths were not scientists but innovators. They were two unusual people who came together because of difficult world circumstances. They could have been the folks next door. They faced all kinds of adversities, had a unique personal affection for each other, and were able to share specific knowledge and experience that came to be widely accepted in the professional world of rehabilitation. They were inseparable throughout their busy careers and in their twilight years. Their concepts about managing and treating children with disabilities, however, will be carried on long after their demise in 1991.

Berta Ottilie Busse was born in Berlin, Germany, on Dec. 5, 1907. Growing up in Germany through World War I, Berta and her family suffered through the difficult times with poor economic conditions, political changes, and anti-Semitism. Berta was interested in gymnastics and wanted to be a gym teacher. She often participated in the activities of the Jewish Youth Club, and it was there that she met Karel Bobath. "We were friends," Berta recalled, "and we went in and out of each other's homes in Berlin." Nothing romantic came of the friendship in those days.

Berta took lessons in gymnastics from 1924 to 1926, with training in normal movement, exercises, and relaxation. "We were taught about the analysis of normal movements and various ways of relaxation. We learned to feel and evaluate degrees of relaxation not only in tight muscles but its effect on the strength and activity of their antagonists. This was done by a special way of handling a person, inducing movements in response to being moved," she recalled. She was hired as an Instructress of Gymnastics at the school but lost her position in 1933 when the school was not allowed to keep a Jewish teacher on staff. For a brief period, she was in Prague and Moscow, later working in London on a visitor's permit. In 1938 she received permission to leave Germany and, because of her training in remedial exercises, obtained employment at the Princess Louise Hospital for Children in London, England.

Karel Bobath was born in Berlin on March 14, 1906, the son of Orthodox Jewish parents. Karel enjoyed the sports activities at the Jewish Youth Club. He often watched Berta. "Berta was a beautiful girl. I sent her notes by way of her younger sister, but it was calf's love. We were frightfully young, and I didn't have much to offer, so we parted."

In 1925, Karel started medical school. By 1932 he qualified as a doctor of medicine. Political undercurrents were stirring, social changes were developing, and anti-Semitism was on the rise. When Karel requested permission to settle in Berlin as a physician, he was denied. He moved to Prague and became a Czech citizen. He learned the language and successfully passed his examinations. After leaving Prague, he worked at a children's hospital in Brno, where his interests centered on pediatrics and pediatric surgery.

In the Beginning: Berta and Karel Bobath

When Czechoslovakia succumbed to Germany's military might in 1938, Karel realized it was no time for a Jewish doctor to remain in Brno. He decided to emigrate to London, England, in 1939. Karel was not admitted to England as a physician. "I was very sad," he recalled. "I had no job and didn't even have permission to study. Things were bleak; life was difficult and depressing."

One morning in 1941, he received a phone call that was to change his life. It was Berta. She had been trying to find him. The Princess Louise Hospital for Children had named Berta chief of the physiotherapy department. One of her patients, the Consul of Afghanistan, was looking for a doctor who would take a job in his country. Berta thought Karel would be willing to take the job. However, when World War II started, Karel discovered that he could remain in London and work as a casualty doctor. His new job at Wilson General Hospital in London allowed him to practice his true profession and help in the war effort.

Berta and Karel were together again, and on April 23, 1941, they were married in a simple wedding.

The Bobath Approach was discovered in 1943. According to Berta, "It was quite by accident." Berta was privately treating a well-known portrait painter who had had a stroke. "Instead of doing what I had been taught," she said, "I observed the patient. Slowly, by trial and error, by observation and deduction, I began relating things he was doing in response to what I was doing. It worked better than anything before." Berta developed her theory during the next 18 months. She found that by stopping her patient from assuming abnormal positions, she was able to reduce his spasticity and help him create new patterns of posture and movement. The patient recovered. He changed his painting style, using his left hand instead of his right, and became even more successful as a result of the changeover.

After that experience, Berta and her physician-husband found themselves becoming interested in the treatment of children with spasticity. They believed early diagnosis was essential in helping to reduce the effects of the condition on the child.

In 1950, Berta took and passed the examination for a diploma in the Chartered Society for Physiotherapists. By 1951, the Bobaths established their first treatment facility in London, where they applied their Neuro-Developmental Treatment to children with CP. Seven years later, they were welcomed to the United States on a lecture/demonstration tour that took them from New York to Seattle. The interest in their treatment regime grew rapidly, and they were invited by professional associations and medical facilities to lecture and teach their techniques internationally.

In 1954, Berta applied for a Fellowship in the Chartered Society. She prepared a manuscript titled "Abnormal postural reflex activity in patients with lesions of the central nervous system" and used it as her thesis. The material later was published as a book in 1965 and has been reprinted in eight languages. It was the first of numerous articles and books the Bobaths authored.

When discussing the treatment approach, Berta always recognized Karel for his support and major contribution. "I did not know that what I called relaxation was in fact inhibition, until much later when my husband became interested in what I was trying out empirically. I want to thank him for the great contribution he has made in explaining the neurophysiological background to my observations, which made the treatment teachable."

With enlarged facilities in London, the Bobaths invited therapists from all over the world to spend several months learning how to treat children with CP. These trained professionals then established programs in other countries and formed The International Bobath Alumni Association to set standards for training and to offer continuing education programs.

"The name Neuro-Developmental Treatment (NDT) was my idea," Berta said. "I am a rather shy person and listen too well to what other people say very often. I was told long ago that treatment shouldn't have the name of the originator, though everybody else calls the treatment by our name. If it shouldn't be Bobath, it should be neuro-developmental treatment. I coined the phase." Berta did hope the name Bobath would be put in brackets after NDT.

By 1989, when interviewed in their home in London, the Bobaths were pleased to note that the Neuro-Developmental Treatment Association (formerly The International Bobath Alumni Association) now had a membership of more than 4,000 professionals. Berta said, "I still can't believe it. It is a dream. And to have the feeling that I have so many friends and good colleagues who will do their very best to continue with it and not let it deteriorate."

During their careers, the Bobaths received much recognition and many awards throughout the world. They received the Harding Award in London for their distinguished work on behalf of disabled children. Sargent College, Boston University, granted Berta an honorary doctorate in humane letters. In 1977, Buckingham Palace invested Berta as a Member of the British Empire (MBE), an honor given only to special people who have given unusual service in Great Britain. Ironically, after having been forced to leave their homes in Berlin before World War II, the Bobaths also received recognition from Germany in March, 1976, when they were awarded the Officer's Cross of the Order of Merit of the Federal German Republic, for "promoting research and medical treatment for children in Germany."

In the Beginning: Berta and Karel Bobath

On April 3, 1991, Peter Bobath, Berta's son, was asked to contribute some personal thoughts to the Bobath biography. Peter wrote, "The memories of those early days were, even then, of their working nonstop on the development of their treatment, the arguments about it, the battles with local authorities to get patients, the disappointments, and the moments of success. The first clinic was then set up, followed by the formation of the charity, now the Bobath Center. In my view, it was a very tough path to choose, which few would have taken up initially and with which even fewer would have persevered. Their working together and love for each other, which was clear to everyone, made the partnership complete. They were, as I remember well, tough parents with strong views, but love was there and, gradually, over the years, I understood them better and better. My tribute is to the early days which must have been the most frustrating, battling, and difficult—yet they won."

Photo by Phil Weedon, London, U.K. Reprinted by permission.

For more clarification of Neuro-Developmental Treatment (NDT) theory and how it influences therapy for children, see Article 1.2 by Judith Bierman, titled "Philosophy, Theory, and Principles: The What, Why, and How of NDT."

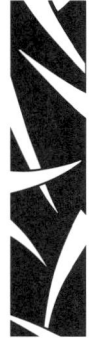

Philosophy, Theory, and Principles: The What, Why, and How of NDT

Judith Bierman, PT

The Neuro-Developmental Treatment (NDT) approach was developed by Dr. and Mrs. Bobath (Karel and Berta) in the 1940s. From the start, they acknowledged it as a "living concept," meaning that the concept would change as understanding of the central nervous system (CNS), CNS disorders, and the needs of the individuals evolved. Over the years, there has remained a very consistent and recognizable approach utilized by a growing number of health-care providers around the world. It is possible to discuss an approach by discussing three major topics: the philosophy, the theory, and the principles. This article discusses each of these topics as related to NDT.

NDT Philosophy

A philosophy is a value system or set of beliefs that unites a group of people. Typically, these beliefs are broad and therefore not possible to prove or disprove. The philosophy that is the base of NDT has remained relatively stable across time. The following statement, developed by the Neuro-Developmental Treatment Association (NDTA), serves as a basic summary of philosophy.

> The NDT approach is a "living concept." It is a problem-solving approach that involves the management of movement dysfunction and the treatment of individuals with CNS pathophysiology. The person is addressed as a "whole," and the intervention process is individualized. The NDT Approach is an interactive process among the involved individual, the caregivers, and the interdisciplinary team.

The overall goal of management and treatment is to enhance the individual's capacity to function. To reach this goal, the therapist addresses the quality of movement by utilizing principles of movement. Intervention involves direct handling including facilitation and inhibition to optimize function. The treatment process includes the gradual withdrawal of the therapist's direct input, leading to increased independence and an enhancement of the quality of life.

What does this mean to you as a parent? A therapist who is using the NDT approach will follow these guidelines:

- The therapist will establish functional goals based on your input.
- The therapist will plan a treatment that treats your child as an individual, important person, taking into account the child's age, personality, problems, strengths, family culture, etc. Therefore, your child's treatment will be different from every other child's treatment.
- The goal of treatment will be to help the child function more independently. The therapist also will spend a great deal of time working on the quality of movement, which refers to "how" the child computes a task. This takes into account the smoothness, efficiency, and ease of performance.
- The therapist will use very special ways of handling or moving your child to help him or her learn to do tasks alone. The handling might include helping the child with movements, doing some movements with the child, or holding the child while he or she moves. Eventually, the therapist will cease handling the child and allow him or her to do the movements and tasks alone.

The basic philosophy has stayed relatively constant throughout many years.

NDT Theory

A theory is a collection of ideas or assumptions that explains a complex approach. The theory may be broken down into smaller assumptions that can be tested in research. For these reasons, the theoretical assumptions for NDT have changed dramatically across the years.

Some of the key theoretical assumptions identified by the NDTA are summarized as follows:

1. The way a person does a task involves the interaction of the person doing the task, the environment in which it takes place, and the specific aspects of the task. In addition, therapists understand that the person is influenced by all of the different systems (muscles, bones, lungs, heart, hormones, nerves, etc.). No longer do therapists view the body as a robot under the total command of the brain.

2. It is important to study carefully how children typically develop and learn how to move. The therapist can apply lessons from this study in planning treatment for children with movement problems.

3. Children with cerebral palsy have some expected difficulties which, if not addressed, can lead to additional problems or secondary difficulties (impairments). All of these problems lead to functional limitations.

4. Treatment begins with a careful assessment (evaluation) and problem solving of what a child can do and how he or she does it. Treatment focuses on increasing functional independence.

These are some of the key theoretical assumptions utilized by therapists who follow the NDT approach. This type of thinking guides the problem solving of therapists who use this approach.

NDT Principles

Principles are the rules that guide the therapist in how to put the philosophy and theory into practice. You might observe your child's therapist following the key NDT principles:

1. Approach the child as a whole, recognizing that the person is more important than the body and considering:
   a. all the systems in the child's body
   b. the entire body during all activities
   c. the environments in which the child typically functions
   d. all the relevant areas of function
2. Individualize intervention according to the child's:
   a. unique movement problems
   b. personality, family, and culture
3. Include assessment in every treatment by constantly observing the child's responses and changing treatment based on those observations.
4. Have the child be as active as possible during every treatment.
5. Use handling as a way to improve the child's function.
6. Use the child's typical environment (furniture and wheelchairs) to work on function, and use therapy equipment (balls, bolsters) to develop movement components needed to complete functional tasks.
7. Use guidelines developed from the study of motor development across the life span.
8. Apply principles of motor learning, and use guidelines from the study of motor control.
9. Use a team approach to treatment.
10. Provide activities for the child's caregivers to do daily so that therapy is not a separate set of exercises but a key part of improving functional activity every day.

What makes NDT unique is not the individual statements in the philosophy, theory, or treatment principles. There are many other approaches that might share some or many of these thoughts. What makes NDT unique is the blending of all of these elements and how you, your child, and your therapist bring these ideas to life.

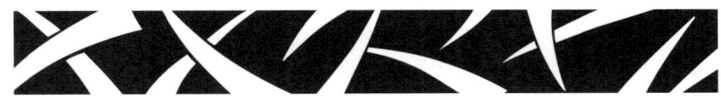

Section 2

Social/Emotional Aspects

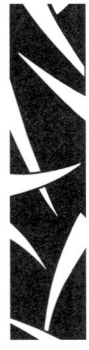

The Emotional Aspects of Having a Child With Disabilities

Suzanne M. Davis, RPT

Parents of children with special needs can find themselves on paths of many different emotions. Many parents talk about feeling great sorrow as well as great joy. These feelings can change who they are and their perspective on life.

I am a physical therapist, a teacher, and, most importantly, the mother of a child with cerebral palsy. I was a pediatric therapist and teacher long before my son was born. Having him has changed my life but ultimately for the better.

I have learned a lot through my experiences and those of other parents whom I have been blessed to know. I wish to share with you some of the things parents might go through. Each parent's experience is unique. As a unique person with a unique child, you might relate to some of this information.

Many parents describe their initial sense of being on a roller coaster. Their emotions move up and down quickly and unexpectedly, depending on how their child is doing. This is especially true of families whose babies have an extended stay in the hospital. There is a sense of being out of control. One minute the baby is doing well. The next minute, things are not going well. The parents feel helpless.

If a baby has to stay in the hospital, the parents become aware that there is a risk of later problems developing. In most cases, even when there is no extended hospitalization, it is the parent (usually the mother) who suspects something is wrong. She notices that her child is not doing the same things as other babies the same age. Or she might have had other children before and realizes that this baby is doing things differently. This is a very scary time. On the one hand, the parent has suspicions; on the other hand, she really doesn't want them confirmed.

When the doctors make a diagnosis, some parents go into shock. I remember going to have tests done on my son for a growth in his belly when he was about 3 weeks old. The doctor came out after the scan and said, "Well, when you're dealing with cancer…" I was devastated. The baby I had waited for so long had this terrible disease. I went into shock. I know that I continued to speak with the doctor and probably even appeared to be listening, but it was like being on automatic pilot. I didn't really hear anything more after the word *cancer*. In fact, I was so out of it that I couldn't even find the five-story garage where I had parked my car, much less find my car! I wandered around for quite a while.

Therapists and doctors wonder why parents don't listen to them. "Doesn't the parent know what's wrong with the child?" Well, if the information is new and emotionally upsetting, parents might not be able to listen because they have shut down inside.

After the diagnosis and the initial shock, parents might experience denial. Sometimes this takes the form of bargaining, thinking things like, "I can accept that my son has cerebral palsy if he walks funny, but please just let him walk." "I can deal with a physical disability, but don't let my daughter have any learning problems." These reactions are common and actually part of the normal process of acceptance.

Another form of denial is seeking other opinions. Some professionals criticize families who do this, but again it is part of the healing process. We might not be happy with the information we've been given, so we look for someone who will tell us that everything is okay.

Guilt is another common feeling that parents have. "Did I do everything I could?" "Did I do something wrong when I was pregnant?" "Could I have done something to prevent this from happening?" (My son's brain injury resulted when he stopped breathing after the surgery to remove his tumor.) We feel guilty over other things as well. Many parents say they feel that they aren't doing enough for their child, such as following the home therapy program more closely or spending more time with their child. They might feel guilty about the time they spend with their child with special needs, because they don't have enough time for their other children or their spouse.

Anger is another powerful emotion that parents sometimes experience. "Why me?" "Why my child?" We sometimes direct this anger at many people and in many places, even at those who are innocent bystanders! I took my son for professional photos when he was about 8 months old, and it didn't go very well. The photographer didn't know what to do with a baby this age who couldn't sit up or hold up his head. I decided to try again when he was about 12 months old. I went to the same studio for the appointment but was told that we weren't on the schedule. I became angry and fought with the woman at the counter, certain that I was right. I was furious. I got back into my car and cried. The anger I felt was strong, but was it really over a miscommunicated appointment time? No, my real issue was that nothing could be normal for me and my son, not even getting his picture taken.

The Emotional Aspects of Having a Child With Disabilities

Somehow, we need to help people understand that we are feeling great frustration and anger and are venting on whoever is in our path at that moment. Our anger is not really directed at that person whose words or actions are just "the straw that broke the camel's back." It might help to explain how we are feeling and ask the other person not to take it personally, but just to listen and be supportive.

Grief also is part of the process. We feel great sorrow about the loss of hopes and dreams that we had for this child. We feel sad when our child is sad. We also feel grief each time we receive a new piece of bad news. This can start the whole grieving process again.

We also might experience the loss of some friends. We might find that friends or family members withdraw because they don't know what to say or do, just like many situations in which people are diagnosed with cancer. This can be very hard for parents because it happens when we most need support.

Acceptance can be a long process but there are two parts to acceptance:

- Our acceptance of this child for who he or she is, because it is so important for us to bond with him or her, love that little person—that spirit that is our child—and build the parent-child relationship, which has a great effect on development.
- Our acceptance of the disability, which helps the child to accept and feel good about himself or herself.

For most parents, the acceptance of the disability takes much longer. Some parents say this will never happen completely for them. We need to realize that it's a different process for everyone. Parents come to terms with the disability in their own way and their own time. The *how* and the *when* are very individual. Remember that acceptance doesn't mean giving up hope.

Although all of these emotions sound hard, there also are many joyful moments and silver linings. The experience of living with your unique child can help put things into perspective. Parents come to realize what truly is important in life. We might be forced to slow down and take life one step at a time. We learn to appreciate the little things in life. Small steps become great joys. We find that we and others learn a lot about unconditional and pure love from our children. In fact, this particular child, no matter how disabled, can change the world and can affect the decisions others make just by being a part of their lives. For example, a cousin of such a child might decide to go into a medical field, a therapist might learn the meaning of patience, or a physician might learn about compassion. These are powerful lessons!

Therapists trained in Neuro-Developmental Treatment (NDT) have a principle that guides them in working with families. That principle is that parents and other family members are important team members. The parent is the expert in regard to the child.

Here are some suggestions that follow this basic principle and can help you through this life process:

- Live each day one at a time. Thinking too far into the future can be very frightening. It is impossible to predict anyone's future. No one knows for sure what any child's ultimate outcome will be. Enjoy your child today, in the moment.

- Ask your therapist to give you ideas for home activities that will help you bond with and enjoy your child as much as possible. Ask for this before you get a set of formal exercises. Do fun, playful things with your child. Don't do a home program when you or your child is not in the mood.

- Make friends with other families who have children with special needs, as well as families who have children without disabilities. Home visits from your therapist can be nice, but they are isolating. Go to the clinic for some of your therapy appointments. Ask your therapists for the names and phone numbers of other families in similar situations. There's nothing like having the support of friends who have been there and understand what you're going through. Create a network of other families for you and your family.

- When other people stare and ask questions, it's very tempting to get mad, but don't. It will be better if you stay relaxed and give a simple, matter-of-fact answer. My son had casts on his legs to stretch out his tight ankle muscles. People asked, "Oh dear, what happened? Did he break both of his legs?" I answered simply, "We're stretching out his muscles." That satisfied them. Everyone was happy. Don't feel that you must give a big explanation and the whole story. It isn't necessary. Now my son does the same thing. He's been asked, "What's wrong? Why do you have that walker?" He answers, "Nothing is wrong with me. I just have cerebral palsy, and I use my walker to walk." Bravo!

- Ask for and accept help. If you always seem to be the main person responsible for the child, ask your spouse to come to a medical appointment with you or to help by doing some of the home activities. Be specific and tell other members of your family exactly what you need. Sometimes a break is the best gift of all! Talk to your therapist about including your other children in therapy sessions. Therapists can design many home programs to incorporate siblings. It doesn't always have to be you. Some of us are so used to doing everything! When strangers offer to help, accept it. For example, let them open the door for you or hold something while you're getting your child into the car.

- Surround yourself with team members who:
  - listen
  - are supportive, compassionate, and caring
  - don't pass judgment
  - answer your questions thoroughly and don't appear to be in a hurry
  - acknowledge you as the expert on your child
  - seem to look for opportunities to empower you
  - have a positive outlook for your child, believe in your child, and share your hope

When you ask a professional for an opinion, you should receive all the possible information. The professional should be honest and open without dashing your hopes. When you make your decision, the professional should respect you for making the decision that is best for your family and should support you even if you are not taking his or her advice. If that doesn't happen, you might want to look for someone else.

Have a sense of humor as you go on this journey. Humor can be very healing and healthy. Many times when we parents appear not to be doing well, it's because we are just trying to survive, doing the best we can at that moment. Be gentle with yourself and encourage others to do so. Be open to all of the possibilities that your unique child can bring to you and the world.

For more clarification of Neuro-Developmental Treatment (NDT) theory and how it influences therapy for children, see Article 1.2 by Judith Bierman, titled "Philosophy, Theory, and Principles: The What, Why, and How of NDT."

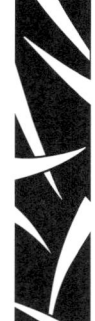

Coping: Movement Made Meaningful

G. Gordon Williamson, Ph.D., OTR

All parents want their children to grow and develop motor skills that give them a sense of achievement and confidence as they interact with other children. Motor skills aren't developed in a vacuum but while children are learning to play and manage other daily activities. Movement becomes meaningful when it helps children cope with their feelings and desires to control objects in their surroundings. For example, the ability to pinch the thumb and index finger together (pincer grasp) becomes significant when a child wants to pick up a piece of cereal, open a milk carton, or button a shirt. Developmental skills such as the pincer grasp are the building blocks for growth.

Coping is the process of bringing together and using those skills in the context of everyday living. Some children aren't successful when they try to cope. For example, some children have only a limited number of coping strategies, and they use them over and over despite the fact that these tactics don't work. Other children have an unpredictable, erratic coping style. They don't have a purposeful plan, and they use their coping strategies in an unsystematic, trial-and-error manner. Still other children have trouble deciphering the demands of a stressful situation. They produce coping strategies that are essentially meaningless because they miss the target.

This article describes the coping process and suggests ideas for you to help your child adapt, especially when reinforcing therapy programs designed to improve motor development, motor learning, and motor control.

Coping is the process of adapting in order to meet personal needs and to respond to the demands of the environment. Children cope with personal needs when they manage their thoughts (e.g., thinking about scheduling for a busy day), emotions (e.g., learning to handle anger), or their physical bodies (e.g., learning to walk). Children also cope with their physical and social environments (e.g., crossing the street safely or sharing toys with playmates). Young children have to manage many new experiences, from trips to a shopping mall to enrollment in a child-care center. They use coping strategies in order to feel good about themselves and their place in the world, especially in situations they interpret as threatening or challenging.

Coping isn't restricted to children dealing with difficult circumstances, however. Most people experience stress as a threat, a negative thing. However, stress perceived as a challenge can be positive, stimulating creative emotions. For example, children working hard to complete new puzzles are coping with feelings of curiosity, a sense of discovery, and strong motivation. In other words, they are coping with challenge. In reality, much of life is a combination of coping with threat and challenge. The toddler looks down a short flight of stairs with an intense desire to go down independently (challenge). However, the same toddler has fears of being hurt in the process (threat).

Coping Resources

A child with sufficient coping resources is better able to manage the demands of daily living, master new learning, and generate feelings of self-esteem. It is important to understand what resources are available to each child and the impact of those resources on that child's perception and management of life events.

Internal resources include:

- beliefs and values
- physical and emotional status
- developmental skills
- coping style

External resources include:

- human support
- material/environmental support

Therapists, teachers, and parents who use the Neuro-Developmental Treatment (NDT) approach can access these resources as they create and modify treatment programs. For example, programs usually are successful if they reinforce children's positive beliefs:

- a sense of trust and security
- an expectation of success and not failure
- an orientation that the world is predictable and reliable
- a sense of personal control

Some children have real difficulty coping. Their coping behaviors can be limited, rigid, or inconsistent. For example, coping with a new baby-sitter might cause some children to withdraw, others to cry, and others to cling to their parents. Children with more flexible coping behaviors might be interested in the stranger and accept the parents' leaving with little discomfort. Children with special needs (developmental delay or disability) seem to react more strongly to the stresses of daily living, which means that they might have problems coping. Some of these children do face a greater number of stresses with fewer coping resources.

It is understandable that many parents of children with physical disabilities focus on their child's motor problems and limitations in movement and posture, which require a great deal of attention. However, a group of well-known child development experts with a broad view of children and their futures developed a list of what they considered the most important abilities that contribute to lifelong success, particularly in school and the community. These critical skills deserve special attention in early intervention, school, and therapy programs:

- confidence
- curiosity
- self-initiation
- self-control
- social relationships
- communication
- cooperation

Current principles of NDT emphasize the development of motor control for function. But it is important also to remember that function implies the use of skills as the child copes with the demands of daily living. The following guidelines can help parents and therapists work together on skill development and adaptability at the same time. For example, a child who is learning to sit with a straight back on the floor can feed dolls together with another child (gaining a motor skill while learning to cope with social and language demands).

- Encourage a good fit between the child's coping resources and environmental demands. When demands and expectations are appropriate to the child's ability to meet them, the child is successful and has a sense of well-being. Overexpectation can lead to placing unrealistic demands on the child and therefore possible failure. Underexpectation can result in low demands that don't motivate the child. Inconsistent demands can cause the child to feel confused and insecure. Parents and professionals can achieve a just-right challenge by (a) modifying demands to match the child's capabilities, (b) enhancing the child's coping resources, and (c) providing accurate and timely feedback to the child's efforts.

- Balance the use of indirect as well as direct intervention strategies.

    Indirect intervention strategies influence the child's behavior through management of space, materials, equipment, and other people in the surroundings. Direct intervention strategies influence the child's behavior through specific interactions the child has with the adult (e.g., physical handling, modeling, verbal guidance). Most children need a combination of direct and indirect strategies. Overreliance on direct intervention strategies can reinforce a passive, dependent coping style. In contrast, the child might be able to perform in a self-generated manner if indirect strategies set the stage for independent functioning.

- Bear in mind the stages of learning: (a) the child first acquires the skill, then (b) becomes fluent with that skill, and (c) carries that skill over into other settings. A child needs to practice the skill in a variety of situations to make sure it is well established and available when needed, even during the stress of daily activities.

- Understand the distinction between a skill acquisition deficit and a performance deficit. A child with an acquisition deficit has not learned the skill for some reason. A child with a performance deficit has learned the skill but fails to use it. The skill might be masked due to anxiety, poor motivation, fear, hyperactivity, or other factors that interfere with performance. Don't assume that the child hasn't learned the skill just because the child doesn't perform it. Examine the factors in the child's environment that could be undermining the child's behavior.

- Encourage the child to take the lead in initiating activities. Some children with disabilities tend to be passive and overly dependent on therapists, teachers, or parents who feel the need to take a rather dominant, lead-taking role. The adult's goal is to elicit responses from the child that the adult then reinforces. Overuse of this pattern can cause the child to become passive, inattentive, or defensive. On the other hand, adults can help the child learn to cope and develop when they expand and extend rather than prescribe and control the child's activity. By responding to the behaviors initiated by the child and encourage turn taking, adults provide support of more self-initiated coping behaviors. The child then might improve his or her ability to express feelings more appropriately, anticipate events, express likes and dislikes effectively, demonstrate per-sistence during activities, and apply learned behaviors to new situations.

- Teach the child a variety of coping strategies.

    Some coping strategies are action oriented to deal directly with the cause of stress. For example, a child who is struggling with a difficult homework assignment becomes frustrated and gives up. Another child with better coping resources might use action-oriented strategies to cope specifically with the task by rereading the instructions, asking a parent for help, or calling a classmate to clarify the assignment. Each of these efforts is focused on accomplishing the homework.

Other coping strategies are emotion oriented to manage the associated tension. These strategies help to energize the child and reduce frustration. The child struggling with homework could take a break, have a snack, or ride a bicycle as means of reducing tension in order to be refreshed for the work. Children need to learn to use both action-oriented and emotion-oriented coping strategies.

Summary

The more effectively a child copes, the more effectively a child learns. A child's coping competence is determined by the match between needs (demands) and the availability of resources to manage them. Successful coping reflects sufficient resources for handling the demands of daily life. Research suggests that coping affects academic achievement, self-esteem, and a sense of personal mastery. Children benefit the most from therapeutic interventions such as NDT when the adults around them understand and reinforce the children's coping styles.

For more clarification of Neuro-Developmental Treatment (NDT) theory and how it influences therapy for children, see Article 1.2 by Judith Bierman, titled "Philosophy, Theory, and Principles: The What, Why, and How of NDT."

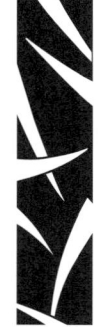

The Autonomic Nervous System: Support for Life

Cynthia Lewis, Ph.D., PT

From the moment we're born, our body's job is to maintain our heart rate, respiration, body temperature, metabolism, digestion, and elimination. These are processes that continue until the moment we die. We often take for granted the influence of these functions on our performance of self-care, academic, and recreational activities.

Our basic body functions are under the control of the autonomic nervous system (ANS), which provides the underlying support for higher order skills such as movement, speech, and cognition (thinking). Homeostasis is the ability of the body to regulate and maintain these functions within a controlled range.

The ANS has a speed-up gear or mode and a slowdown gear or mode. The speed-up mode is the sympathetic nervous system (SNS), and the slowdown mode is the parasympathetic nervous system (PNS). You might have heard the SNS referred to as the fight-or-flight mechanism. This mode is associated with a "hyper" state of alertness; stress (actual or perceived); anxiety; excitement; intense emotions, such as fear, anger, or joy; quick, hurried movements such as running, jumping, or flailing of the arms; and pupil dilation. During times of stress, some people experience rapid heart and respiration rates, nausea, and a cold, clammy feeling. These are signs of the SNS mode.

When a child is upset, crying, or stressed, the SNS speed-up mode dominates. Parents easily recognize crying as a sign of stress but need to realize that other stress signals include hiccups, spitting up, a wide-eyed expression, hands and feet in the air as if pushing away, bluing of the skin, turning the head away, flailing of the arms and legs, kicking, or even falling asleep. A very active, moving child also is in more of a speed-up mode and under greater SNS influence. The heart and breathing rates are faster and energy expenditure is higher.

As you might guess, the PNS generally has an opposite effect from the SNS. The PNS is associated with a calm or sleep state, rest or low level of activity, slow or normal heart and respiration rates, and digestion. The sleeping child, under greater PNS influence, is in more of a slowdown mode. Heart and breathing rates are slower, and energy expenditure is lower. When eating or sitting quietly and playing, the child is in a combination of both SNS and PNS modes, balancing each other. In this quiet, alert state, heart and breathing rates are moderate and energy expenditure is at a low to moderate level.

Muscle activity also causes changes in the ANS. If the child sees a toy and reaches or crawls toward it, arm, leg, and trunk muscles have to work. Those working muscles use more energy, so they signal the brain to increase SNS activity, which in turn increases heart and breathing rates to get oxygen and fuel to the muscles. Once the child has the toy and is playing quietly, the muscles are working less and have a lower demand for oxygen. Then the muscle signal to the brain is to increase PNS activity, which in turn decreases heart and breathing rate. Thus the brain constantly adjusts heart and breathing rates to meet the oxygen need of the muscles for current energy expenditures.

Because SNS and PNS modes not only affect a child's behaviors but also are affected by a child's activity levels, we can plan activities that change modes to help modify those behaviors. Activities that change the child's behaviors can aid the child in changing states or level of alertness. Table 1 describes methods to enhance SNS or PNS activity. Note that the activities are almost opposite of each other for stimulating or enhancing the two systems.

Enhancing SNS	**Enhancing PNS**
1. Bouncing the infant or child	1. Bundling in a blanket
2. Posture with arms and legs extended or away from the body	2. Posture with arms and legs bent or flexed close to the body
3. Louder music and voices	3. Softer music and voices
4. Interrupted noises	4. Constant sounds like a fan, car engine, or vacuum cleaner
5. Bright lights	5. Soft or dim lighting
6. Cooler temperatures or bath	6. Warmer temperatures or bath
7. Moving surfaces such as rolls and balls	7. Stable surfaces such as bed or sofa
8. Sitting up	8. Lying down
9. Movement	9. Being quiet and still
	10. Sucking a thumb or pacifier
	11. Eating, chewing, or drinking

Parents and caregivers already use many of these activities to help their infant or child become more calm or alert. For example, parents often help infants to calm themselves by using a pacifier, which enhances the PNS or slowdown mode. They discover that moving or bouncing the baby quickly can turn on the SNS or speed-up mode and help the baby become more alert in preparation for social interaction. In general, activities that decrease breathing rates will activate the PNS, and those that increase breathing rates will enhance the activity of the SNS. By improving your skill at reading your child's cues, you then can use the PNS-enhancing activities in Table 1 to help your child develop self-calming and self-regulation skills.

Control of basic body functions is essential in order to perform higher functioning activities or skills. For example, to sit alone with trunk control in order to use the hands for play (higher order function), the child has to breathe (basic body function) without having the movements associated with breathing cause a loss of balance. Even we as adults tend to hold our breath or breathe shallowly if our balance is challenged when walking on ice, for example.

Researchers have shown that infants born prematurely or with neurological impairment have more difficulty regulating the actions of the ANS than infants born full-term and without impairment. These infants expend a great deal of energy just to maintain body functions such as regulating and maintaining heart and breathing rates and body temperature. Less energy is available for staying awake, interacting with caregivers, and moving arms and legs. Because the lungs are immature in the very premature infant, the energy cost of breathing and even just expanding the chest can be significant, requiring much more energy than for the adult.

The energy cost of movement also is greater in a child with a neurological disorder, such as cerebral palsy, Down syndrome, or spina bifida. Because of muscle weakness, these children have to make their muscles work harder than do their peers to perform the same task. An increase in muscle-work effort increases the oxygen demand, which places a greater demand on the heart and lungs during movement. Thus, these children fatigue more quickly than children without impairment. Weakness in abdominal and chest muscles makes chest expansion and inhalation more energy costly than for other children. Changes in position and posture affect breathing. When the child is lying down, gravity assists inhalation. When the child is sitting up or standing, gravity assists exhalation. You can help your child's breathing by altering the child's position and posture during an activity. For example, to use gravity to assist with inhalation, place a child with limited postural control in an inclined position.

Neuro-Developmental Treatment (NDT) Principles

You can apply NDT principles of intervention to everyday life, as outlined below, to help these children achieve a balance of the SNS and PNS—a quiet state of alertness for optimum learning.

- **NDT Principle:** Parents and other caregivers are important members of the team.

  Activity: Parents providing interactive supportive care

  Method: Help develop self-consoling skills by holding the infant's or child's arms and legs bent and cuddled against yourself or bundled in a blanket. Encourage the baby to suck on his or her hands or thumb to learn self-consoling skills.

- **NDT Principle:** Development of skill acquisition relies on the child's integration of interaction of his or her body's multiple systems, the task, and the environment.

  Activity: Maintaining balance in any posture, as in sitting for play

  Method: Grade the intensity of the activity so that the child can do the task with a minimal to moderate energy cost. Support the child as much or as little as necessary to accomplish the task of sitting and to expend low to moderate energy so that arms and hands are free for play activities. In supported sitting, you'll need to stabilize the trunk not only for posture and activities, but also for chest expansion and deep breathing that will support a balance of SNS and PNS.

- **NDT Principle:** Learning occurs during goal-directed activities that are motivated by pleasure.

  Activity: Manipulating toys in different postures for integration of postural support necessary for movement skills

  Method: Place toys at different heights on the floor, on a low stool or bench, on a sofa, and on a table. Have your child climb, reach, squat, crawl, roll, and stand to get the toys. Place toys so as to challenge your child's skills but still allow success.

- **NDT Principle:** Distal mobility (arm, hand, and finger movement) depends on active or supported stability of the head and trunk.

  Activity: Balancing on a large therapy ball

  Method: Provide as much support as necessary at the hips/trunk while shifting the child's base of support from side to side and forward and backward (Figures 1a and 1b) to challenge sitting balance and improve trunk control for balance and respiration.

The Autonomic Nervous System: Support for Life

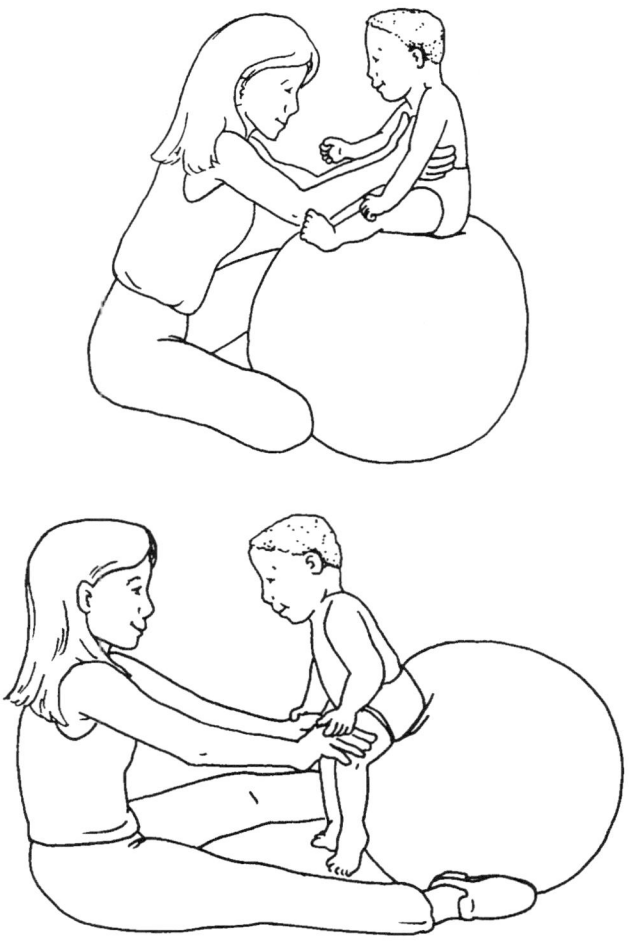

Figures 1a and 1b. Shifting base of support forward.

Summary

You can challenge your child to develop new skills with just-right tasks that minimize stress to the child's systems. Activities in Table 1 can help children learn self-calming or self-alerting techniques. Children who can handle stress with minimal energy cost will have more energy for learning new skills and participating in activities, and will be less fatigued at the end of the day.

For more clarification of Neuro-Developmental Treatment (NDT) theory and how it influences therapy for children, see Article 1.2 by Judith Bierman, titled "Philosophy, Theory, and Principles: The What, Why, and How of NDT."

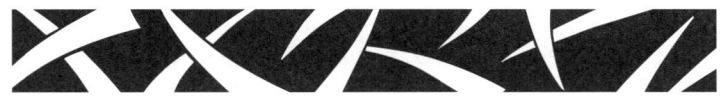

Section 3

Posture and Positioning

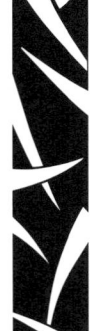

Postural Control: Stability for Function

3.1

Barbara Cupps, PT

Sit up straight! Many children have heard this from their parents and grandparents. Maintaining good posture is important so that we don't grow up with a crooked spine or rounded shoulders. Traditionally, young girls practiced walking with books balanced on their heads to improve their posture.

What Is Posture?

Posture is more than a straight back. It is the alignment of body segments to each other and their position in space. For example, a flexed posture of the arm indicates that the elbow is bent. A stooped posture in standing is a combination of many parts: rounded shoulders, forward head, rounded back, and bent hips and knees. Posture varies depending on a person's position and the activity the person is performing. The ability to assume and maintain postures is called postural control.

Karel and Berta Bobath, who originated the Neuro-Developmental Treatment (NDT) approach, studied normal postural control and the problems children and adults with neurological impairments have with posture. They emphasized the need for efficient postural control in order to perform skilled movement. Much of their treatment was based on minimizing atypical patterns of postural control and obtaining more efficient postures and patterns. Alignment and coordination of posture with movement are still important concepts of current NDT treatment principles.

Many factors influence posture. Gravity is one of the primary external forces acting on the body. Body segments are naturally aligned to oppose this force. Bones, joints, ligaments, tendons, and muscles provide stability to the body. When postural control is efficient, the musculoskeletal system has mechanical stability. That is, each segment is balanced upon the one below (like stacked blocks). Therefore, the person exerts only a minimum amount of muscle activity to remain upright. The spine, for example, has a natural S-shaped contour. This is efficient for stability in an upright position against gravity and yet allows mobility for movement.

Some parts of the body always are in contact with a supporting surface. This is called the base of support. Only in a weightless situation (such as in space) is this support unnecessary. The body parts are aligned from this base of support to counteract the force of gravity. In standing, the base of support is the feet. Postural activity of the foot and calf muscles helps to maintain the legs upright over the feet; hip, spinal, and abdominal muscles keep the trunk erect over the legs; neck muscles maintain the head so that the eyes are horizontal (Figure 1). Erect posture is the result of both muscle activity and stability from bones, joints, and ligaments.

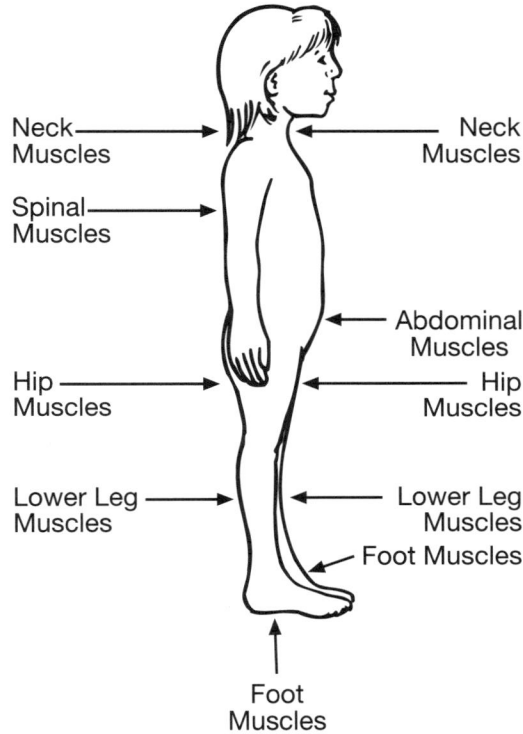

Figure 1.

Gravity isn't the only force acting on body parts. Internal forces result from muscle action and the movement of body segments during activity. For example, momentum is built up during the forward movement of the legs during walking. The individual must accommodate these forces in order for movement to be smooth and coordinated. Thus, walking requires additional muscle activity to slow down the forward movement of the legs, counteracting and controlling the forward momentum.

The mechanisms that control posture are extremely complex. We use sensory information to determine relative positions of our body parts and the forces acting on them. We need knowledge of the functional activity to be

Postural Control: Stability for Function

performed and stability requirements for that task. Trial and error are important for learning postural control.

Types of postural control include balance reactions, postural preparation, and stabilization during movement.

- Balance reactions act to prevent a fall. Falling is the result of body segments being out of alignment so that gravity pulls the body toward the ground. Vision, input from the inner ear, and sensory information from the joints and skin tell the brain when you are beginning to fall. You correct posture through muscle activity, which realigns the body segments to prevent falling. Sometimes, this involves catching yourself with your arms. Other times, it means righting body segments, returning to a stable position. Sometimes, postural reactions aren't quick enough and you fall.

- Postural preparation enables you to stabilize the body segments, change a base of support, or change alignment before movement begins. This helps you perform an activity efficiently and successfully. These preparations for movement often are called *postural sets*. Activating trunk and leg muscles before pushing a heavy object is a postural set or preparation. Placing arms in a supporting position or placing the feet farther apart are examples of changes in postural set before beginning an activity.

- Stabilization of the head, trunk, and limbs occurs during movement. For example, muscle activity in the hips and trunk takes place as you reach forward with the arm. Reaching in a limited space requires the trunk to maintain its stable position. Reaching farther away requires the trunk to follow the arm, which requires a weight shift over the base of support. Postural activity of the muscles allows just the right amount of shift without falling.

Postural control develops from birth and continues throughout life. In the early months, a baby gains control of the head and trunk with the help of external stability. For example, Mom and Dad support the baby yet allow the head to bob and the trunk to get erect. With some external limits, the baby learns to control the alignment of body parts. As development continues, the child explores limits of internal control. For example, a 7-month-old who is beginning to sit independently on the floor will reach for a toy. If the baby reaches too far, the child loses his or her balance. The first time, the baby might fall. The next time, the child might catch him- or herself with the arms. With repetition and experience, the child learns automatic postural control specific to that activity.

Children with neurological impairments often have great difficulty developing postural control. A child who is "floppy" (hypotonic) doesn't have enough stability to support upright posture and movement. A child who is stiff

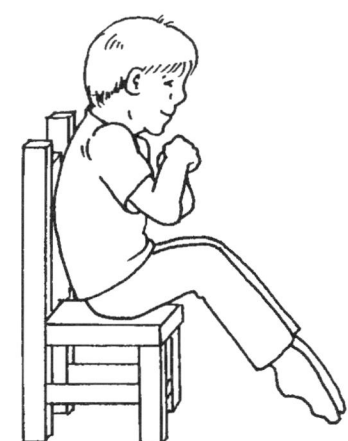

Figure 2a.

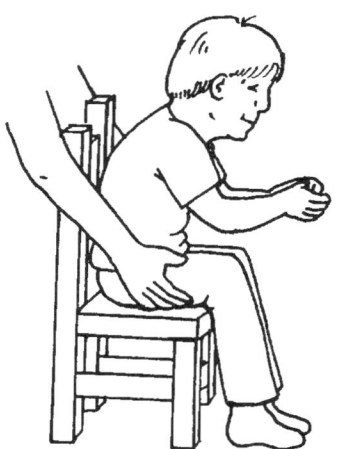

Figure 2b.

(hypertonic) often uses that stiffness for stability but can't change it for a movement or postural response.

You can help your child utilize more efficient posture for a task. One way is to help align the body parts so that the child is more stable for a particular activity. For example, a slouched position in sitting makes reaching forward difficult (Figure 2a). The child is sitting with most of the body weight back in the chair, and the spine is rounded. Without adjusting this posture, the child will be able to reach forward only in a limited range. It is difficult to extend the arm and turn the hand up to grasp. When the child bends the hips and brings the trunk forward, then he or she is able to hold the trunk and head erect and reach forward (Figure 2b). Try this yourself. Sit in a chair, lean back, and slouch. Pretend you are reaching forward for a glass of water, but don't change your posture. Now come forward to sit tall and see how reaching is so much easier.

Postural Control: Stability for Function

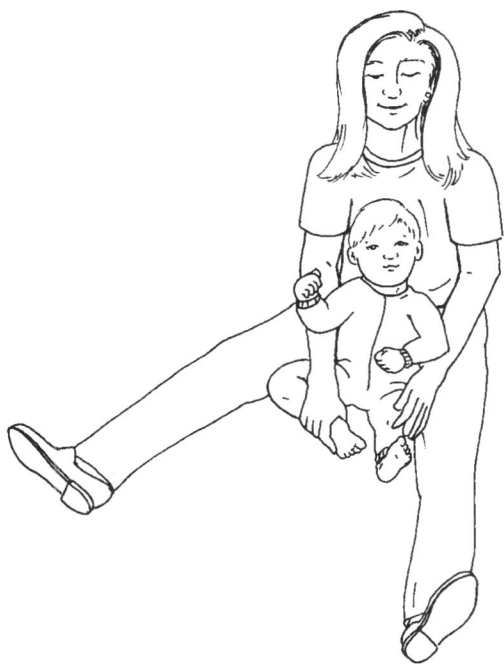

Figure 3.

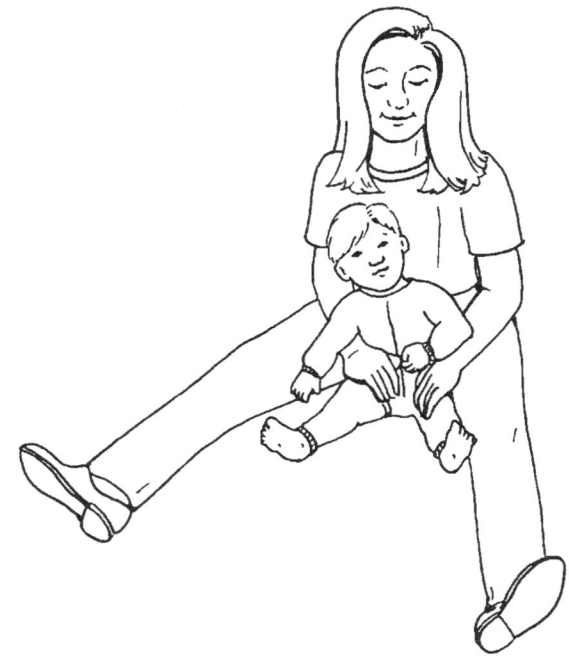

Figure 4.

A base of support can provide varying amounts of stability and mobility. You can adjust or change the child's base of support to make posture or movement more efficient. A wider or larger base of support is more stable than a narrower or smaller one; however, mobility over that base of support is more limited. Sitting with the legs apart can be very stabilizing for a young child. However, it is more difficult in that position to reach to the side or to move out of sitting. Moving one foot in, closer to the body, makes it easier to weight shift to that side (Figure 3).

Providing external stability limits is another way to help your child learn postural control. Sit on the floor and place the child between your legs. Use your arms around the child's trunk to narrow the surrounding space (Figure 4). You may apply slight pressure down on the legs (the base of support) so that they are active in postural control. Don't fully support the child, and allow some movement of the trunk. If the child falls into your arm, wait for a righting response (the child moves off of your arm back to upright). If the child doesn't respond, slightly lift your arm to facilitate the action. Gradually withdraw your arms as the child begins to gain more control.

Controlling the alignment of all body parts during functional activities is difficult and complex. Children with stiffness often become more stiff as they try to do things because they can't coordinate the control of so many parts. You can help by controlling one or more parts and allowing the child to control what he or she can. Figure 5 shows a child bringing a toy to his mouth. The mother supports some of the weight of the arm and helps the elbows bend. The child is active in holding the toy as well as controlling the head and trunk.

Equipment also can provide assistance in postural control. Chairs and seating systems ideally provide alignment and stability limits for a child while allowing active postural

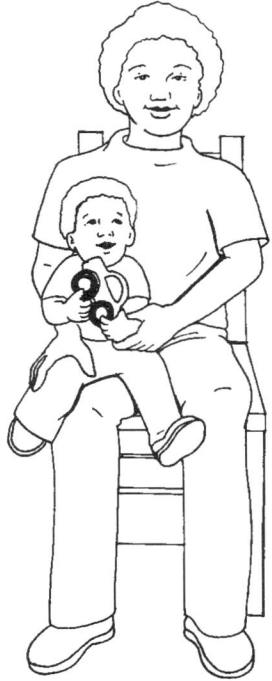

Figure 5.

control. A tray on a wheelchair can provide upper-extremity support to assist in head and trunk control. A contoured seat supports the hips and buttocks more than a flat seat. Standers allow a child to be upright, actively supporting weight through the legs and feet. A walker provides more stability than canes or crutches.

Precautions

Active postural control requires a great deal of energy for some children. Watch for signs of fatigue: loss of head or trunk control, falling, or irritability. Give your child more support or change position for a time.

Make sure your child is safe. When learning postural control, children can lose their alignment easily. Be ready to give them more support if they need it. It's okay to let them lose their balance if they can catch themselves with their arms or if you are going to break their fall. Place pillows around a young child on the floor to provide a soft surface on which to fall. Use safety belts when needed. Check with your therapist regarding specific ways to help your child increase his or her level of postural control.

Summary

Postural control is necessary for maintaining an upright position and orienting the eyes and ears to the environment. It is also needed for moving in the environment and for hand function. For the child with postural-control challenges, equipment and/or handling can help by (a) establishing a base of support and alignment, (b) narrowing stability limits, and (c) controlling or supporting some body parts.

Give the child the opportunity to develop and use the maximum active postural control of which he or she is capable. You can help your child get upright, stay upright, and move!

For more clarification of Neuro-Developmental Treatment (NDT) theory and how it influences therapy for children, see Article 1.2 by Judith Bierman, titled "Philosophy, Theory, and Principles: The What, Why, and How of NDT."

Quality of Movement: The Importance of Postural Control for Functional Activity

Linda King-Thomas, M.H.S., OTR/L

Most children with cerebral palsy, even those mildly affected, have significant problems with postural control. These problems are obvious when they try to move from one position to another or try to use their hands. They might lose their balance or need to use their hands and arms for balance, and as a result, they have difficulty playing with toys or feeding themselves.

Because postural control involves sensory components as well as motor (muscular and skeletal) components, a child with cerebral palsy also might have difficulty organizing and adapting sensory information about a certain object, learning from past experiences (feedback), and using that information for a similar but not identical object. For example, a child might not be able to transfer the skill of drinking from a lidded cup to drinking from an open cup. Anticipation of the new action (feedforward) might interfere with coordination. In fact, just thinking about it might cause increased muscle stiffness.

Why is postural control so important, especially for the child with cerebral palsy? Everyone needs to organize the motor components as well as the sensory components of postural control in order to solve the problems of carrying out everyday activities. For example, when I reach for this toy, how far can I shift my weight before I fall? How fast do I tip this cup with no lid so that I can drink but not spill my juice? Postural control provides a stable base from which the child can perform functional activities.

This article will help you understand the motor and sensory components of postural control. This understanding can help you train your eyes to become expert at identifying your child's needs and strengths. You then can do your own problem solving about the most appropriate positions of postural support for your child during play, where to place hands on your child to support posture, and ideas for activities to develop postural control.

Muscular and Skeletal Components

Postural control, which develops in the first year of life, is necessary to be able to move in a world where gravity exerts a constant force. The muscular and skeletal components of posture include antigravity movements of flexion (bending) and extension (straightening), rotation (turning or twisting), weight shift, structural alignment, and balance reactions.

The young infant gradually develops muscle control against gravity to raise the head, sit up, and stand. When both flexor and extensor muscles of the trunk become strengthened and balanced, the infant becomes able to rotate the trunk. If the extensor muscles are stronger than the flexor muscles, only limited rotation can develop, and movement is inefficient and poorly coordinated. This happens to children with cerebral palsy.

All movement involves a weight shift and rotation, sometimes a very small amount (reaching for a toy while lying on the stomach) and sometimes very large (moving from the stomach to sitting or standing). Rotation allows movement to occur in a three-dimensional plane. All of the transitional movements (going from one position to another) include rotation: rolling, sitting to hands and knees, back lying to sitting, sitting to standing, climbing into a chair, and rotating to sitting. The balance of flexion and extension muscles, weight shift, and rotation results in smooth, fluid, and coordinated movements.

Structural alignment is another component that is important for efficient movement. One way to evaluate the structural alignment in the body is to observe the symmetry of body parts (shoulders, trunk, hips). When a neuromotor insult to the nervous system (such as cerebral palsy) affects postural control, maintaining alignment during movement becomes a challenge. It is important for both therapists and parents to learn how to use their hands during therapy and home activities to help the child maintain body alignment for more efficient movement patterns.

Righting and equilibrium reactions (which affect balance) also are very important for the development of postural control. Righting reactions involve the orientation and alignment of the body in space. Equilibrium reactions are balance reactions in response to an external disturbance that shifts the center of gravity. For example, if a child is bumped by another child and the center of gravity shifts too far for recovery (equilibrium reaction), a protective reaction might occur in which the child extends an arm forward, sideways, or backward, depending on the direction of the displacement, to prevent the body from falling. If righting and equilibrium components of postural control aren't well developed, the child tends to rely on the arms to maintain balance in sitting or standing. As a result, the arms are less available for play, exploration, finger feeding, and other daily life activities. Until the child develops adequate postural control, adaptive equipment such as specialized seating, side supports, and chest harnesses can help free the child's hands for play and self-care activities.

Sensory Components

The sensory components of postural control include information from many systems: visual, vestibular (gravity and balance information from the inner ear), proprioceptive (data from muscles and joints about the position and orientation of the body), and tactile (touch). Other components are anticipatory postural adjustments (feedforward) and the development of sensory pictures of one's body in the brain (feedback). Feedforward is information telling the body what to do to get ready to move. Feedback is information that tells the body what the movement just felt like.

The visual, vestibular, and somatosensory (tactile and proprioceptive) systems provide information to the child about the position of his or her body in space.

The visual system provides information about the vertical plane by observing vertical objects in the environment (walls, people standing).

The proprioceptive and tactile sensory systems provide information about the muscles and positions of the trunk, head, arms, and legs, as well as characteristics of the supporting surface (hard floor, grass, soft sand).

The vestibular system provides information about the pull of gravity and the balance reactions needed when there is a change in the center of gravity for the current body position. When a child loses his or her balance, the center of gravity shifts. The vestibular, proprioceptive, and tactile sensory systems then provide information to the central nervous system for regaining the lost balance and bringing the center of gravity back to the centered position. This sensory information plays a critical role in the development of feedback and feedforward mechanisms involved in postural control and skill development.

Feedforward is an adjustment in posture the child makes in preparation for movement. As the child anticipates the need to reach, grasp, catch, kick, or throw, the various receptors of the eye and inner ear stimulate the changes in posture and movement the child needs to complete the task successfully. The type of anticipatory adjustment depends on the child's past experiences with the particular activity and the materials and spatial arrangement of the task. Parents and therapists can evaluate the status of anticipatory postural control by observing the quality of these preparatory motor actions.

When a child with cerebral palsy anticipates engaging in an activity such as eating or playing, the brain relays feedforward messages to the postural system. These messages frequently result in an increase of muscle tone, stiffness, and possibly rigidity even before the child has started the motor activity. You will need to recognize the role of anticipatory feedforward messages and their effects on an impaired postural system. You then can prepare the child through positioning and/or handling techniques even before the child receives visual or auditory input. For example, securely position the child in a stable chair in a calming environment before you mention lunch or present food.

The feedback mechanism, which develops first and provides information to the brain both during and after a motor action, plays a critical role in the learning process and has a significant impact on postural control. The sensory information gained from the experience of being touched, being moved, and moving independently shapes a picture of the body in the brain. As the child grows, the feedback sensory information continually reshapes and updates this picture of the body in the brain.

Feedforward control develops closely behind and in parallel with feedback control. Information about the body gained from sensory feedback becomes the basis for anticipatory feedforward information, problem solving, and skill acquisition.

Through visual, tactile, and proprioceptive sensory feedback, the child learns how far the arm needs to move in order to reach a cup, how the hand needs to be shaped to pick up the cup, and how fast to tip the cup when drinking to prevent spilling. As the cup-drinking skill emerges, the anticipatory feedforward information becomes part of the problem-solving process of reaching, holding, and drinking without spilling. Anticipation of the postural and motor actions of a task allows for quicker, more automatic, and more efficient execution of the task. Then, when an open cup replaces the lidded cup, feedback and feedforward provide refinement of all this sensory information, and managing a new cup becomes a successful problem-solving process!

Practice and Repetition

Practice and repetition are important in developing the anticipatory postural control needed for problem solving and skill development (learning). During practice and repetition, the nerve pathways in the brain become more efficient and feedback/feedforward mechanisms have many opportunities for ongoing refinement.

In addition, active participation, rather than passive movement, is important for learning because the thinking process of anticipating a new action activates the feedforward mechanism. Active participation includes both the sensorimotor action and the emotional investment (motivation).

It is important to remember that the child needs to experience both success and failure in learning a skill. The sensory feedback from the success or failure is an essential part of the learning process and contributes to future problem solving. For example, if the child never experiences the weight shift and displacement of the center of gravity when falling, he or she won't know how and when to make the postural control adjustment needed to regain balance. All children need to experience a variety of directions and speeds of movement. This broad sensory information base is necessary for development of anticipatory postural control responses and problem-solving movement patterns needed for specific skills.

How does postural control help the child? It provides a stable base of control for functional activities to occur.

If the trunk and shoulder girdle are stable, then the arms can move skillfully in the daily activities of play and self-care (feeding, dressing). As the arms develop control and stability, the hands and fingers can learn delicate fine-motor patterns such as the pincer grasp for small-object play, buttoning, zipping, and using a pencil.

If the trunk and pelvic girdle (hips) are stable, then the legs and feet can move in efficient patterns for walking and running. Coordinated movement in the arms, hands, and legs also requires the postural control components of movement against gravity, rotation of body parts (internal and external rotation), structural alignment, and balance and equilibrium reactions (foot equilibrium reactions, orientation of the arm in space, protective extension reactions).

Neuro-Developmental Treatment (NDT) principles provide useful guidelines for therapists and parents involved in home programs:

- Skill acquisition relies on the interaction of the body's systems (sensory, motor, emotional), neural maturation, and interaction with the environment.
- Learning occurs during goal-directed activities that are motivated by pleasure.
- Postural control appears to be learned and modified with experience—both success and failure (feedback and feedforward).
- Key points of control (hand placement) assist in the execution of efficient and coordinated movement.
- Parents and other family members are important members of the team.

Suggested Activities

Therapy ball

Using a therapy ball is an excellent way to develop postural control. Gently bounce the baby on the ball in a seated position to help prepare the muscles of the trunk for the holding and moving patterns described here:

- You can encourage your child, seated on the ball, to use rotation to cross the body midline with one arm while reaching for desired objects. Place the object high or low, near or far, keeping your hand(s) at the child's hip(s) during rotation and/or reaching to the side.
- You also can use the therapy ball to encourage extension against gravity. As your child lies on his or her stomach with your hand supporting the hips, encourage the child to reach for a favorite toy and play in this position. Try placing toys on a bench or coffee table to get the correct height in relation to the therapy ball. Roll the ball forward and backward slightly to help activate the extensor muscles through vestibular input.

Tire inner tube

Sometimes, a movable surface such as a therapy ball can be difficult to control and too challenging for the child. Laid flat on the floor, an inner tube from a car tire (or truck tire for a larger child) provides a great alternative to the therapy ball. It is bouncy like the therapy ball and therefore provides some surface movement, but it is much more stable and won't roll around.

- With the child seated inside the circle, the inner tube provides support to the low back, a confined area, and safety in the event of falling. With the trunk supported, the child's arms and hands are free for play and self-care activities such as feeding. The floor position also encourages play with other children.
- With the tire still flat on the floor, place the child astride the tire (one foot inside the circle, the other outside; see Figure 1 on the following page). Sitting on the tire in this straddle position provides motor challenges for postural control in muscle activation against gravity, structural alignment, weight shift, rotation, and balance and equilibrium reactions. The straddle position also gives the child a wide base of support for stability.

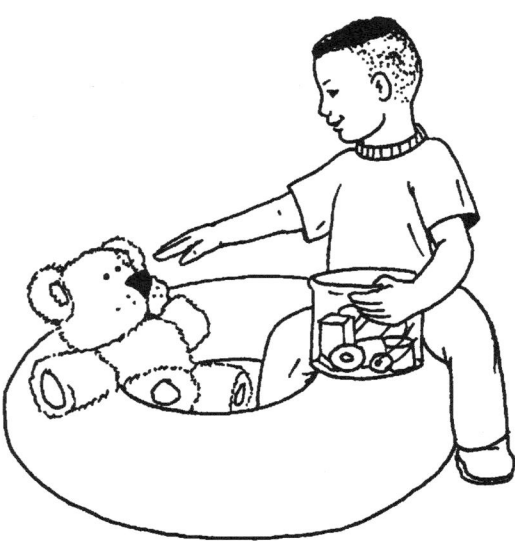

Figure 1. Gently bouncing on the tire activates the muscles of the trunk and prepares them for action. You can place your hands at key points of control (hips, trunk, knees, feet) to assist in the alignment and stability of the trunk.

- Introduce play activities such as playing with shaving cream spread on the tire (which encourages weight shifts as the child reaches out to play with the shaving cream), moving toys from inside the tire to outside the tire (rotation and balance), and reaching for toys that are away from the tire (balance and equilibrium in a higher center of gravity). Pretend that the tire is a lake or a hiding place. The child can climb into and out of the tire to problem-solve the spatial organization of the body in relation to another object (feedforward and feedback).

Pillows and cushions

Place sofa cushions, bed pillows, and large homemade pillows (bedsheets filled with chunks of upholstery foam) on the floor to create a challenging surface for rolling, crawling, and pushing around. The uneven surface provides dips that require flexion against gravity to move out of the "valleys" from back lying. Your child will have to use weight shifts, rotation, balance, and anticipatory planning for the transitional movements needed to navigate the pillows. Active participation in family roughhousing on the pillows will give your child the success and failure learning experiences needed to achieve new skilled movements in the context of play.

Summary

Postural control is a necessary part of learning new skills. It gives a stable base from which mobility for functional skills can emerge. Repetition and practice in a variety of situations give the feedback and feedforward mechanisms many opportunities to receive input for learning and problem solving. Activities that challenge the components of postural control (antigravity movement, weight shift, rotation, balance, and equilibrium) in the context of play (goal-directed and pleasurable) develop the foundational stability and problem-solving strategies needed for skill acquisition.

For more clarification of Neuro-Developmental Treatment (NDT) theory and how it influences therapy for children, see Article 1.2 by Judith Bierman, titled "Philosophy, Theory, and Principles: The What, Why, and How of NDT."

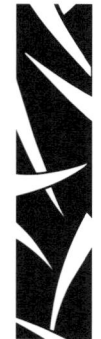

Is W-Sitting a Problem? Managing the Modeling of Bone and Joint Geometry

Beverly Cusick, M.S., PT

Has your therapist or doctor advised you that your child should not use the W-sitting position to play? Are you getting conflicting opinions from different professionals about this issue? W-sitting is a common sitting position for children with diplegic or quadriplegic cerebral palsy if their thigh bones and knee joints have formed in such a way that makes the position comfortable and stable for play. There are two main types of W-sitting: Type 1 (Figure 1), with feet turned out, and Type 2 (Figure 2), with feet turned in. This discussion addresses Type 1 because it can damage the inside knee ligaments, contribute to knee joint instability and dysfunction, and promote chronic knee pain in adolescence and adulthood.

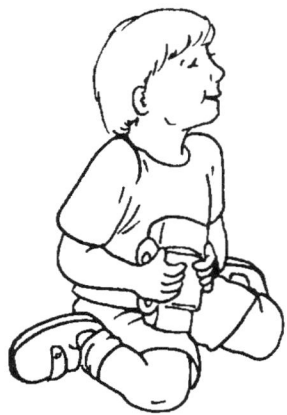

Figure 1. W-sitting, Type 1, with feet turned outward (heels in, toes out).

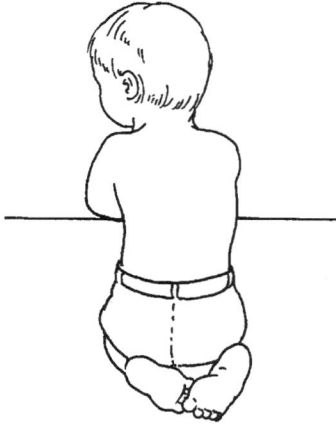

Figure 2. W-sitting, Type 2, with feet turned inward (heels out, toes in).

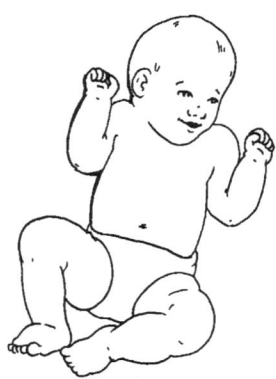

Figure 3. Fetal position: hips and knees flexed, knees apart, feet close together.

How can cerebral palsy influence the shape of the leg bones?

During the last two months of pregnancy, the mother's uterus becomes increasingly confining, bending the hip and knee joints of the growing baby and turning the thighs outward and the legs inward into the fetal position (Figure 3). Shortened muscles at the hips and knees are primary factors in maintaining the fetal position.

After birth, the infant's bones, which are made mostly of pliable cartilage, slowly harden as they gain calcium deposits until growth is finished. During the first 8 years, when the bones are least rigid, many significant changes in bone and joint design occur through a process known as *modeling*. When bone and ligament modeling progresses normally, daily movement activities apply the forces of body weight and muscle pull to growing bones and joints until the mature skeleton suits the functional requirements of adult life. Though some bone shapes are inherited (high-arched feet, for example), modeling changes the shape of bones and joints. Infancy is the time of greatest change in bone geometry due to modeling.

The newborn infant in fetal position hides the normally twisted shape of the femurs (thigh bones) under tight hip muscles. If the hip muscles were not so tight, we might be able to see that the bottom end of the femur is normally twisted inward (medially) about 25° more in the full-term newborn baby than it is in the average adult (Figures 4a and 4b). This twist is called medial femoral torsion (MFT; also

Is W-Sitting a Problem? Managing the Modeling of Bone and Joint Geometry

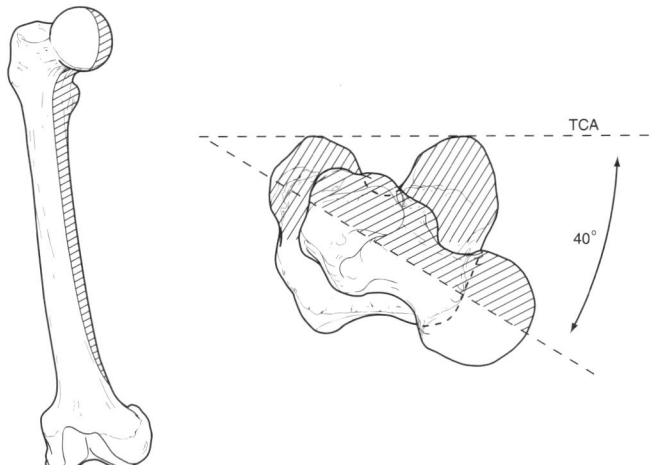

Figure 4a. Newborn medial femoral torsion.

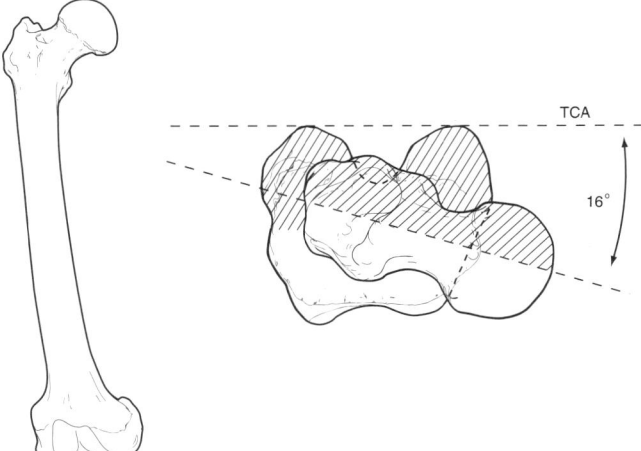

Figure 4b. Adult medial femoral torsion.

known as femoral anteversion). Evidently, the shortened hip-joint muscles and ligaments offer a secure hold to the upper end of the femur so that daily crawling, climbing, walking, and running activities apply thousands of outward rotation forces to the lower femur, gradually untwisting it. Children with cerebral palsy often fail to untwist their femurs fully because they can have any or all of the following:

- weak muscles
- lax ligaments
- few and predictable movement skills
- a body that was born too small to have achieved the size that would have imposed fetal position
- balancing and movement strategies that are immature or that compensate for weakness or problems of muscle control

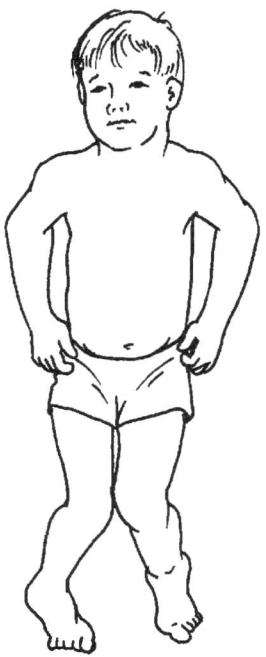

Figure 5. This child with cerebral palsy has weak muscles and rotates his legs medially. His femurs model according to these loading and movement patterns, retaining immature MFT.

These problems can lead to standing and walking with hips and knees bent and thighs rotated medially (inward). The growing femurs apparently sense the persisting medial rotation forces and model accordingly by twisting more medially (Figure 5).

Does W-sitting increase medial femoral torsion (MFT)?

W-sitting doesn't seem to increase medial femoral torsion. More likely, W-sitting is comfortable for children who already have increased MFT because the lower end of the femur is already twisted inward.

So what's the problem with W-sitting?

Have you ever watched an infant move back and forth between all fours and the sitting position? Hundreds of times a day, the child rotates hips to the floor, lowering the pelvis beside the legs and controlling the transition mainly with the muscles of the belly, outer hips, and thighs. If the child sits on the floor with both legs in front of the trunk, you usually will see him or her move to all fours by reaching forward or to the side, raising the pelvis above one bent leg, and transferring weight to that same knee (Figure 6).

Is W-Sitting a Problem? Managing the Modeling of Bone and Joint Geometry

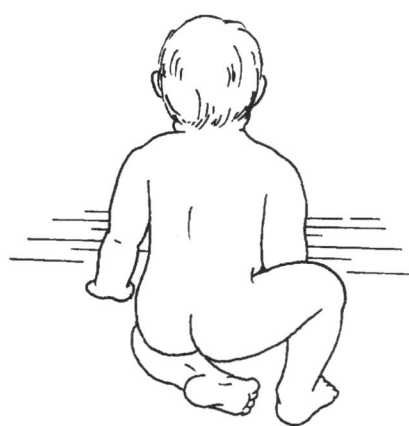

Figure 6. Infants without disabilities typically use this vaulting transition between sitting and the all-fours position hundreds of times every day.

If children who W-sit can crawl or bunny-hop on all fours, they move to sit by lowering the pelvis straight backward and down, between the legs. They don't use the outer thigh and hip muscles. Instead, they repeatedly use the muscles of the low back and of the front and inner thighs.

Muscles also adjust in size and length to the way that they are used most commonly. Infants of 10 to 15 months of age gradually achieve and use long sitting (legs stretched out in front of the trunk; Figure 7) because they lengthen the hamstring muscles on the back sides of their thighs and knees. Children with cerebral palsy, however, usually continue W-sitting, and the hamstring muscles remain shortened. Shortened hamstring muscles pull the pelvis backward (sacral sitting, Figure 8) and make sitting with the legs in front of the trunk too difficult to use for meaningful play activities. The child fails to develop side sitting, long sitting, ring sitting, and tailor sitting, along with the transitions into and out of these positions.

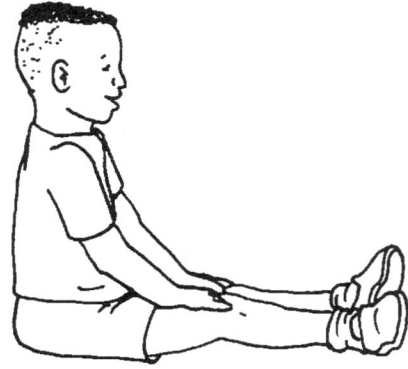

Figure 7. A normal long-sitting position.

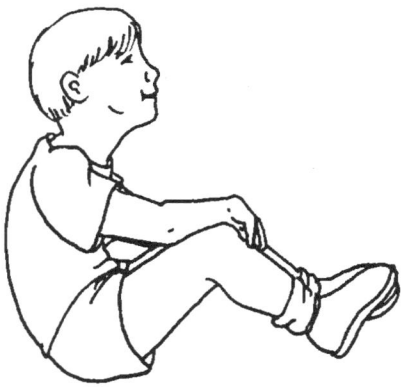

Figure 8. Sacral sitting. Weak back muscles and tight muscles on the back and insides of hips, knees, and ankles make play in this position impossible.

How can increased medial femoral torsion affect my child's walking ability?

Type 1 W-sitting stretches the supporting ligaments on the inside of the knee joints because the floor forces the legs and feet into lateral (outward) rotation. The likely result of persistent W-sitting is postural malalignment syndrome, whereby excessive MFT and excessive lateral twist (torsion) of the lower leg bones (increased tibiofibular torsion) occur together. Postural malalignment syndrome occurs in some children without disabilities who, by the end of adolescence, typically develop knee pain that increases with activities such as skiing and running. Ligament laxity (increased mobility in a joint due to looseness of the supporting tissues) is possibly a contributing factor to postural malalignment syndrome in these children.

The growing child with cerebral palsy also has the problem of weakness and usually stands and walks with the hips and knees bent as well as rotated medially by MFT (Figure 9, following page). The ligaments on the inside surface of the knee joints stretch out, reducing their load-bearing stability. The knees eventually can appear more *knocked* as the child grows taller, and they might hurt in weight-bearing positions as early as 10 years of age. Recent studies of adults with cerebral palsy reveal that many ambulatory adults and teenagers stop walking, either as older teenagers or in their 40s, and that problems with knee pain are common.

Meanwhile, at the bottom of this collapsing system, the feet usually strain into pronation, flattening the big inner arches (Figure 10, following page). Pronated feet are flexible and able to absorb shock forces, but they lack the stability needed to propel the body forward effectively or efficiently. Foot pronation is a major factor in leg muscle fatigue.

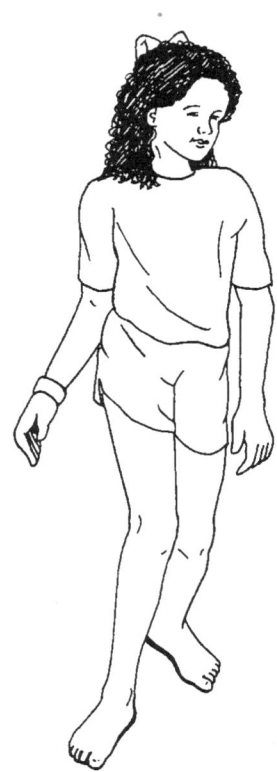

Figure 9. Postural malalignment syndrome. Femurs twist inward at the knee; leg bones twist outward at the ankle.

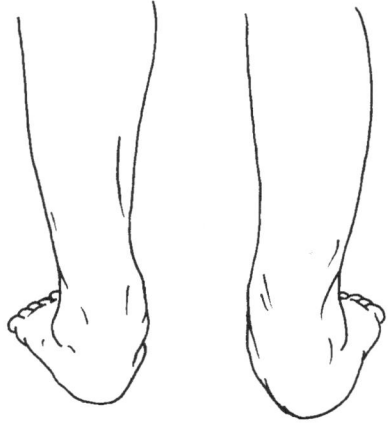

Figure 10. Foot pronation: collapsed arches.

My child is older than 5 years of age. Can Neuro-Developmental Treatment (NDT) correct excessive MFT?

No one knows. In my opinion, if you consider treatment sessions to be professionally guided exercise, undertaken for up to an hour, one to four times per week, then probably not. Bone modeling seems to require several thousands of applications of the proper forces over several years, particularly the very early years. Because the bones in most 5-year-old children have hardened considerably, they are less responsive to modeling forces. However, NDT is like many therapy approaches that not only emphasize the role of appropriate joint and postural alignment for optimum function but also stress the need to integrate therapeutic goals and techniques into everyday activities. Formal studies using reliable X-ray methods to measure MFT before and after a therapy course would help to determine this possibility.

My child is younger than 24 months of age. What can I do to prevent my child from developing postural malalignment syndrome and increased medial femoral torsion?

Orthopedists rarely if ever measure femoral torsion in infants. The radiologic (X-ray-type) techniques are too unreliable at this time. Without this baseline information, we don't have evidence of torsional status as it relates to any therapy approach. Meanwhile, we bring what we understand about bone modeling and muscle actions to a comparison of the leg bone designs of people with and without cerebral palsy. In so doing, we can assume logically that consistent and very carefully selected therapy activities, beginning early in infancy, might help to reduce MFT to some extent. However, if modeling the femur requires 5,000 to 15,000 repetitive rotary forces in weight-bearing positions applied each day, such as walking with a normal pattern of leg movements and alignment, then full correction by handling and therapy probably won't happen. Many factors would have to be considered, such as the child's age and ability, interest in moving, and the frequency of successfully activating the modeling muscles and movements.

The preventable component of W-sitting is the knee-joint laxity and instability and the accompanying increased lateral twist in the leg bones below the knee that commonly result from Type 1 W-sitting.

You might consider the following strategies to address the prevention of rotary knee and leg deformity and at least a measure of MFT:

- If you have read Nancie Finnie's book, *Handling the Young Cerebral Palsied Child at Home* (see References for Parents at the end of this volume), you know to begin by holding your child in ways that will keep the thighs rolled outward and apart. Promote weight-loaded hip lateral rotation and extension (straightening). For example, play "horsey" with your child straddling your thigh or belly, and encourage him or her to stand up and sit down repeatedly while you keep the thighs apart and turned outward (Figures 11a, 11b, and 11c).

Is W-Sitting a Problem? Managing the Modeling of Bone and Joint Geometry

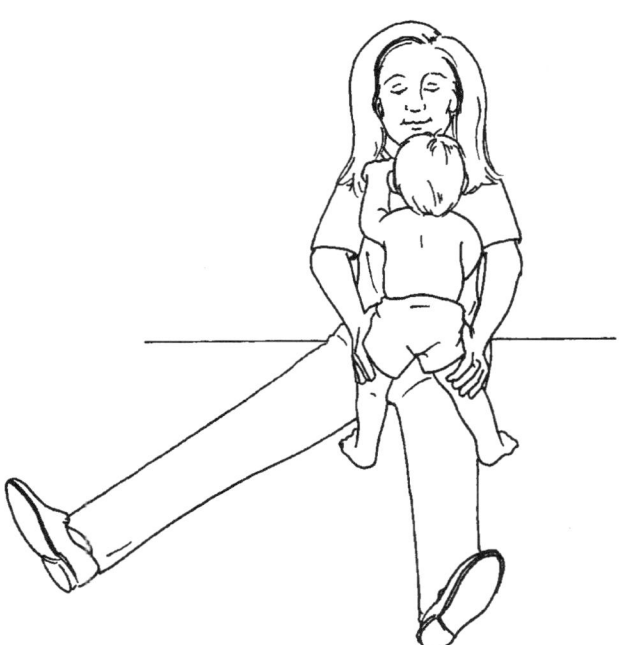

Figure 11a. Straddle sit to straddle stand.

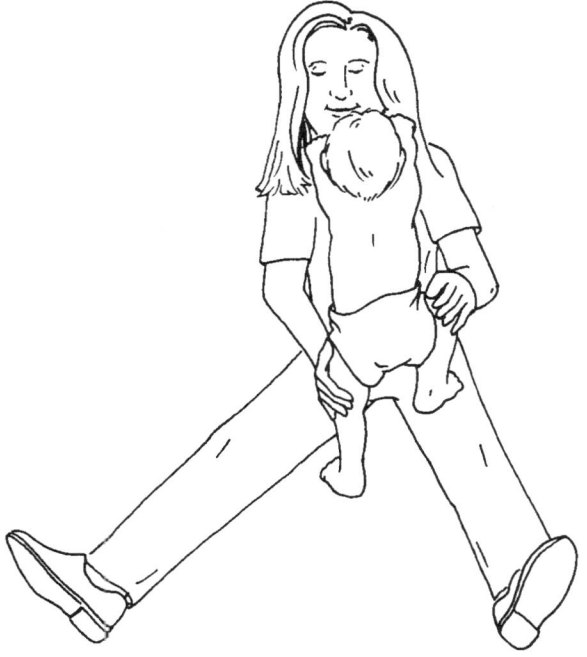

Figure 11b. Weight shift to other leg, keeping knees apart and preparing to climb.

- Stay close to your child and coax him or her to climb up any and all safe objects such as carpeted stairs, sturdy child-sized chairs, big beanbags, piles of sofa cushions, and upholstered furniture.

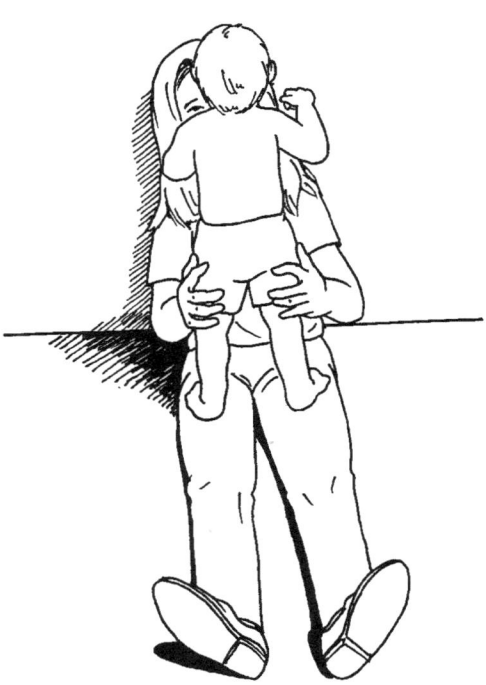

Figure 11c. Repeat on both sides (as long as you still have hair on your head!).

- Keep your child's play position options open. Prevent shortening of the hamstring muscles behind the thighs and hips. Ask your therapist for positioning ideas to lengthen the hamstring muscles.
- Your therapist might try elastic strapping or taping techniques to promote lateral hip rotation or at least to reduce the apparent medial hip rotation, all day long.

Can surgery correct increased MFT?

In the right hands, absolutely. Talk with your rehabilitation team members about the pros and cons of various procedures known as femoral derotational osteotomies (FDROs). Reports in the literature are favorable. Search for an experienced surgeon who is glad to show you his or her outcome data. New surgical methods are much less painful than you might expect, and casting after surgery might be optional for your child. Ask about the protocols for post-operative care, because methods differ widely among physicians and facilities.

If your child W-sits with feet turned inward (Type 2), then an operation to untwist the femurs might be sufficient to improve the overall walking pattern. In the case of postural malalignment syndrome associated with Type 1 W-sitting, however, your surgeon might have to untwist both femurs to correct the medial torsion and the lower leg bones (tibias) to correct the lateral torsion. The possibilities for surgical complications are doubled by the addition of the lower leg bones to the operation. Some surgeons refuse to take the risk, leaving your child with the likelihood of living through adolescence and adulthood with daily knee pain and related limited function. Other surgeons are experienced and capable of addressing all of these alignment issues in one operation.

Does it really matter if I let my child W-sit (Type 1) to play?

Prohibiting your young child from W-sitting is about the future, not the present. If your child is severely involved and unlikely to walk independently, then I would say "no." Your child's independence and freedom to move about and experience some success in a play activity are more important. Try to maintain hamstring length and back muscle strength. However, if your child is a potential walker in the home, school, and/or community, then I would say that W-sitting does matter. Prolonged W-sitting can interfere with functional walking and its pain-free life span.

How do I prohibit W-sitting?

Your therapist can help you to find positive solutions and viable alternatives. Encourage your child to join you in caring for his or her knees, to help them to grow as straight as they can, to prevent them from hurting, and to minimize future surgical needs. Remember, too, that long bone malalignment usually imposes pronation forces on the feet, with its accompanying problems of fatigue (refer to Figure 10).

Strategies for preventing W-sitting that have met with success in various families include the following (this list is by no means complete):

- Most children without disabilities who are approaching 10 months of age pull to stand and cruise along furniture, walls, and crib rails. They also usually spend considerable time standing up. Most children with cerebral palsy remain on the floor for several years, crawling as the main means of moving about. Instead, encourage your child to spend more time in the standing position, cruising along furniture. Move play activities to the sofa or onto an adjustable-height play table, for example. Resist the temptation to use infant walkers to facilitate standing, however, because they are notoriously hazardous and might promote leg movement patterns that are characteristic of a child with stiff muscles.

- For a child with postural malalignment syndrome, forcing ring sitting (with the soles of the feet together) or tailor sitting (with the ankles crossed) is uncomfortable and potentially harmful to the hip and knee joints. Provide a variety of alternative seating and standing options for play, including barrel seats, riding toys, long-sitters, and/or stationary standing devices, if needed.

- See whether your child would accept TherAdapt® Knee Skis (available from TherAdapt Products®, Inc., 800-261-4919) while playing on the floor. These devices prevent the wearers from sitting down between the feet.

- About 3 weeks of tying shoelaces together or of using linky legs might be adequate to help your child find alternatives to W-sitting. Linky legs are fabric-covered neoprene or rubber loops connected with a stretchy strap. Wearing this device on the ankles during floor play keeps the feet from separating enough to permit the child to sit down between them, but the device doesn't impede crawling, kneeling, side sitting, long sitting, or tailor sitting (Figure 12).

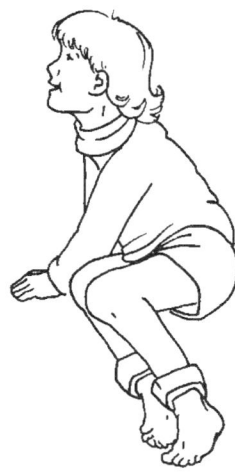

Figure 12. Linky legs for floor play prevent W-sitting, Type 1.

- Taping to promote hip lateral (outward) rotation might quietly deter your child from W-sitting and help you refrain from issuing repeated verbal reminders. This very new management strategy would require tuning to find the optimum fit of the tape such that it works as a reminder not to W-sit, but still is well-tolerated and safe for the skin. Your therapist can attend continuing education courses on pediatric taping.

- If your child does not pull to stand spontaneously while playing, remove ankle and foot braces and shoes if they appear to add outward twist force to the lower leg during floor play. If possible, ask your child's orthotist to design a lock-and-release ankle joint that can allow the feet to point down while the child is playing on the floor. Better yet, find play positions and locations other than the floor.

Is W-Sitting a Problem? Managing the Modeling of Bone and Joint Geometry

Decades ago, Berta and Karel Bobath, the originators of the NDT approach, stressed the importance of early diagnosis and intervention for children with cerebral palsy. They recognized the W-sitting problems and consistently promoted the achievement of hip lateral rotation in their patients. NDT is one of several therapeutic approaches that emphasize the importance of achieving and restoring proper bone and joint alignment as a necessary part of moving efficiently. W-sitting opposes this effort. Your therapist's specialized training can generate a wealth of ideas to help you find satisfying management strategies for your child's optimum muscular and skeletal development.

For more clarification of Neuro-Developmental Treatment (NDT) theory and how it influences therapy for children, see Article 1.2 by Judith Bierman, titled "Philosophy, Theory, and Principles: The What, Why, and How of NDT."

Orthotics/Orthoses/Braces/Splints: What Could They Mean for Your Child?

Allison Whiteside, PT
Illustrations by Steven Whiteside, CO

Your child's physical therapist has said that it's time to consider using an orthosis to help in positioning your child's feet.

Most therapists, including those who use the Neuro-Developmental Treatment (NDT) approach, realize that this effective, hands-on method doesn't exist in isolation. Therapists use NDT with a variety of other modalities, including casts, splints, and orthoses, that sometimes are essential treatment components for some children to achieve alignment, the basis for posture and movement.

So what is an orthosis? Could the therapist be talking about those ugly metal braces or orthopedic shoes or those things that athletes put in their shoes? How will your child like this new thing? Will it be ugly? Will it be comfortable? Will it make your child look different from other children? Will your child really be able to walk in a brace?

What is an orthosis?

An orthosis is a custom-made piece of plastic that puts your child's feet into the best possible alignment and holds them there. The words *orthosis* (single brace), *orthoses* (two or more), and *braces* are interchangeable.

Your physical therapist will discuss the prescription for an orthosis with your child's attending pediatrician. Some pediatricians will agree with the recommendation and write a prescription. Other pediatricians might not feel confident in their knowledge of the feet and will refer your child to a pediatric orthopedic surgeon.

The pediatric orthopedist will complete a comprehensive exam of your child's muscles, bones, and joints in order to have a baseline understanding of your child's spine, legs, and feet development. The pediatric orthopedist then will evaluate your child's feet and legs with respect to orthosis management, talk with the referring physical therapist, and write a prescription.

Next, a certified orthotist will cast your child's feet in the correctly aligned position. The orthotist then uses this cast to make an orthosis agreed upon by the expanded team of physical therapist, pediatric orthopedist, pediatrician, certified orthotist, and you, the parent.

As you can see, your child's team has just expanded by one or two team members. But it takes such a team to get the best treatment for your child.

What is a splint?

Some physical therapists who have taken courses in making splints for the feet and legs might request a prescription for a splint. A splint can help to evaluate what type of orthosis the child might need in the near future, or a series of splints might be used with a young child during the growing years before an actual referral to a certified orthotist takes place. A physical therapist makes a splint out of a low-temperature thermal plastic, draping the plastic on the leg and forming it directly on the leg into the maximum aligned position.

So why does my child's physical therapist want to put orthoses on my child's feet?

The child's feet are the base of support, the part of the body that is the foundation for standing. If the base upon which we stand is out of alignment, the rest of the leg and body also will be out of alignment. For example, some children stand on only the outsides of their feet, on the insides of their feet, or on their toes. If the child continues to stand on only a part of the foot rather than on the entire foot, the foot bones could start to deform. Over time, the deformities get worse because one group of muscles works too hard and another group of muscles works too little. Also, the child who is standing on only a part of the foot cannot feel the entire foot on the floor. Without feeling their feet on the floor, children don't have the confidence to stand alone. The confidence comes from having good balance that results from standing on correctly aligned feet. Therapists sometimes try to prevent deformed feet by putting the child's feet into orthoses or splints before the child begins to stand.

The orthoses put the feet of your child in their best alignment to optimize knee, hip, and body control. With a solid base of support, your child now can feel the floor with the entire foot. Working in standing with your child is a very important goal for the physical therapist. Standing also is important to occupational and speech therapists who might be using standing frames in the child's home and/or school. Aligning the feet in custom orthoses enhances all supported standing.

Sitting balance also depends on the feet being firmly planted on the floor, because the base of support includes the feet as well as your child's bottom on the chair. Without

Orthotics/Orthoses/Braces/Splints: What Could They Mean for Your Child?

the foot support, your child will be working too hard, with muscles out of balance in the legs and/or body, and will feel unsafe sitting alone.

Okay, so now I understand why you want to put my child in an orthosis, but what will it look like and what types are there?

During different developmental stages, your child will need different types of orthoses to support the feet and legs. The long-term plan is to build increasing support in the feet over time. The support comes from the brace and from the correctly aligned muscles, tendons, and ligaments in your child's feet. At some points in development, your child might need maximal support from a brace. At other times, your child won't need an orthosis or will need only minimal outside support. Development of the legs, feet, muscles, and bones changes constantly over time.

Modified Insoles/Footwraps

Most therapists usually begin standing a young infant during therapy sessions between 6 and 12 months of age. The therapist might choose to modify a pair of high-top leather tennis shoes with an insole to diminish the toe-grasping, shift the weight of the body into the heels and onto the outside border of the feet, and create arches within the feet. Or the therapist might decide instead to make a wrap of your baby's feet in a correctly aligned position with a flexible fiberglass material. The therapist cuts the wrap down the middle so you can open it and put it on your baby's foot. You then would need a shoe with an open toe to put over the wrap.

Dynamic Slippers

Once your child begins crawling and possibly pulling up on furniture, your physical therapist might request that your child move into a dynamic slipper (Figure 1). A dynamic slipper is made of a very thin plastic that allows for stability of the foot with some mobility within the orthosis. It is helpful for a child who has good range of movement in the heel cord and needs control only of the joints of the foot.

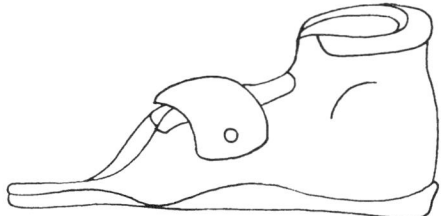

Figure 1. Dynamic slipper.

Supra Malleolar Orthosis (SMO)

At this same time in development, the therapist might recommend a supra malleolar orthosis (SMO; Figure 2) for a child who has the skill of a toddler, crawls to get around, pulls up to stand, and attempts walking around furniture, but has poor control of the foot from side to side when standing.

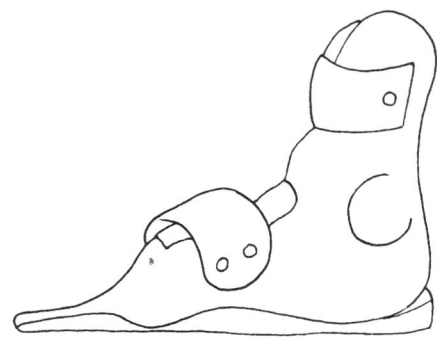

Figure 2. Supra malleolar orthosis (SMO).

Dynamic Ankle-Foot Orthosis (Dynamic AFO)

As your child begins to walk between 2 and 5 years of age, the demands upon the orthoses change, and your team might prescribe a different orthosis. The dynamic AFO (Figure 3) is a very thin plastic orthosis that permits some flexibility between the lower leg and the foot. This orthosis allows the heel to strike the floor with each step yet provides enough stability to keep an elevated heel down. It's also good for children who have strong tightness or low tension in their muscles when they begin a standing program in a piece of adaptive equipment.

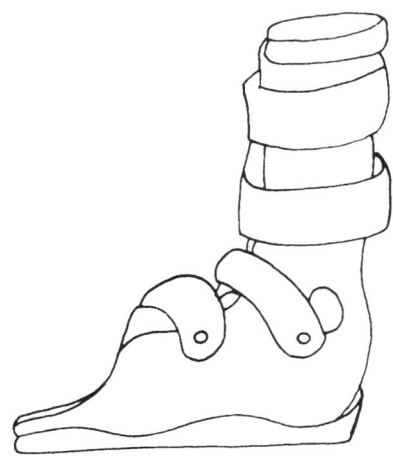

Figure 3. Dynamic ankle-foot orthosis (AFO).

Posterior Leaf Supra Malleolar Orthosis (Posterior Leaf SMO)

Some children new at walking tend to walk on their toes, are unable to strike their heel when walking, or pop their knee back when standing. Your therapist might recommend a posterior leaf supra malleolar orthosis (posterior leaf SMO; Figure 4) to help the child plant the entire foot during the standing part of walking, to control the knee in standing, or to bring the knee over the foot when walking.

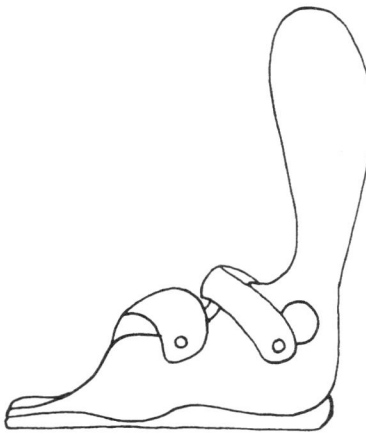

Figure 4. Posterior leaf SMO.

Articulated AFO

Another type of AFO recommended for a child just beginning to walk includes a variety of articulated AFOs (Figure 5). The orthotist builds different types of ankle joints into the system, with "stops" to prevent or assist movements that match the demands of the walking cycle. Physical therapists often request articulated AFOs because they allow the child to move the ankle up or down when walking while preventing collapse onto the inside or outside of the feet.

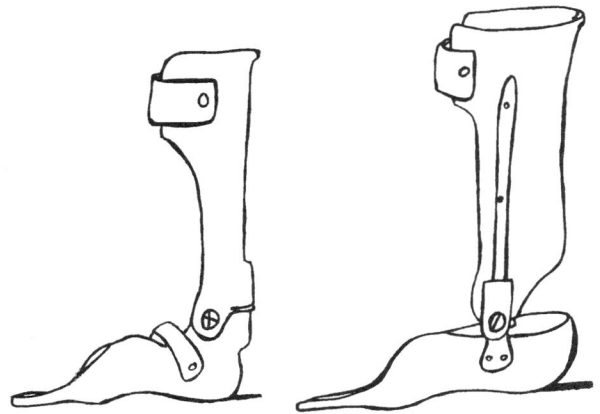

Figure 5. Different types of articulated AFOs.

Solid Ankle Orthosis

Some children might be older when they learn to walk. A child who is learning to walk at 6 years of age or older is considered a late walker. The age of your child, body size, type of muscle tone, and muscle strength are factors that your team considers in deciding what orthosis to recommend. A solid ankle orthosis (Figure 6) might be appropriate because of tightness in your child's heel cord, strong straightening patterns in the muscles of the legs, or a collapse during the standing phase of the walking cycle. The orthotist can make the solid ankle AFO so that it can be converted into an articulated AFO at a later time. Your therapist will be able to predict whether your child might gain enough motor control within the lifetime of the brace so that the manufacturer can make the orthosis convertible from solid (nonmovable) to articulated (movable at the ankle).

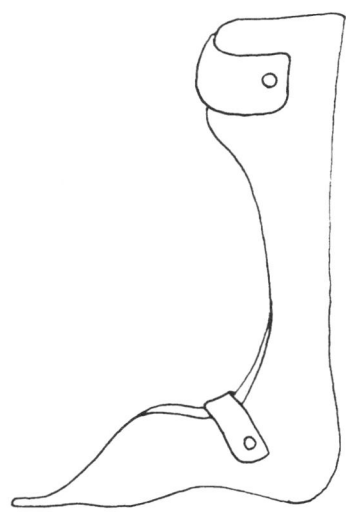

Figure 6. Solid ankle orthosis.

Two-Stage AFO

Another type of orthosis for a child late to walk is the two-stage AFO (Figure 7, page 48), which can capture the difficult-to-fit foot into a dynamic slipper that is then slipped into a more rigid AFO. This orthosis is appropriate for the foot with a lot of tension in the muscles and tendons, the foot with poor sensation, and for the caregiver who has difficulty placing the tight heel into a brace.

Orthotics/Orthoses/Braces/Splints: What Could They Mean for Your Child?

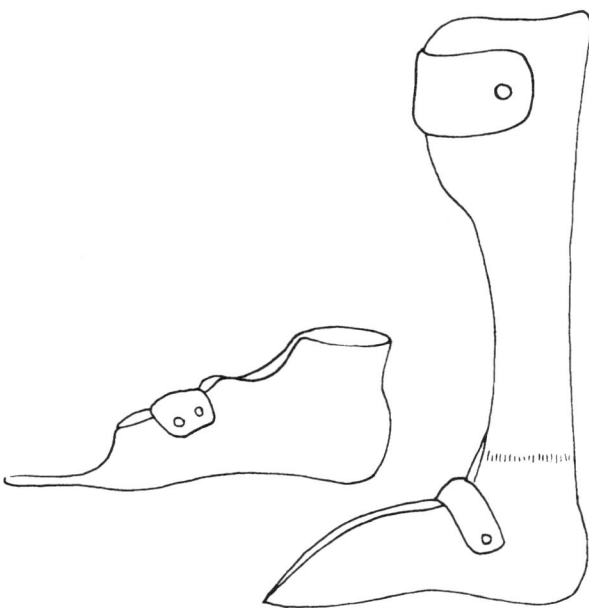

Figure 7. Two-stage AFO.

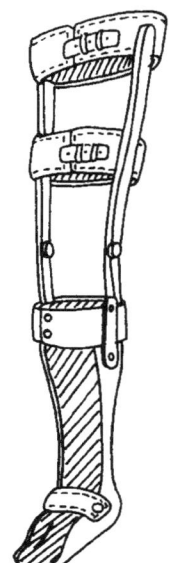

Figure 8. Long leg brace.

Long Leg Brace

Although a major goal for most parents is that their children learn to walk, it is a goal that isn't always achievable. However, even if some children aren't able to walk functionally, standing needs to be a critical part of their days. They might have the long-term goal of being household walkers and assisting with transfers. Therefore, older children benefit from continued orthosis management, such as long leg braces (Figure 8), to preserve the integrity of the structure of their feet, which are maintained from all prior orthosis management. A long leg brace starts with a solid ankle AFO that is connected to metal uprights, always attached to the outside of the AFO, and sometimes to both the outside and the inside of the AFO. The metal uprights connect to the body by a knee pad, thigh band, thigh cuff, and/or a pelvic band. The brace might leave the knees free or strap them into a straight position. Goals of the long leg braces are to place the feet directly below the hips, bring the hips and body over the feet, straighten the hips so that they can go over the feet, straighten very bent knees, keep the muscles of the legs lengthened, and/or begin to teach older children and teenagers to take steps in a walker while wearing the long leg braces.

Now that I understand this developmental perspective of how therapists recommend and prescribe braces over the life of a child with special needs, I'm compelled to ask whether my child will always need braces.

That's a hard question to answer because of the variety of children who benefit from orthosis management. Children typically wear orthoses throughout their growing years. There might be periods of time out of orthoses, but during growth spurts, children might need to resume wearing braces. Your pediatric orthopedist might recommend surgery instead of an orthosis. The surgeon might tell you that further orthoses might not be necessary if your child has the surgery or that orthoses will be critical afterward to maximize the outcome of the surgery. If the team only knew the answer, your decisions as parents wouldn't be so grueling.

Overall, a well-fitting orthosis is your child's friend. It will help your child learn the functional skills of pulling to stand, cruising, walking with two hands held, walking with one hand held, walking alone, running, and hopefully, jumping for joy!

Artwork copyright © by Steven Whiteside. Reprinted by permission.

For more clarification of Neuro-Developmental Treatment (NDT) theory and how it influences therapy for children, see Article 1.2 by Judith Bierman, titled "Philosophy, Theory, and Principles: The What, Why, and How of NDT."

These Arms Are Meant for Reaching: Upper-Extremity Casting for Functional Alignment

Audrey Yasukawa, M.O.T., OTR/L

Many children with cerebral palsy have problems using their hands because of decreased range of motion or abnormal alignment in one or more joints of the arm. Functional joint range in the more proximal joints of the upper extremity is essential for providing the variety of movements the hand needs to work efficiently. For example, a contracture at the elbow can limit the range for extending the arm to reach for a toy. Furthermore, problems with rotating the forearm might limit the ability to orient the hand in space to pick up the toy. Malalignment or instability of the wrist can affect the ability of the fingers and thumb to work together for playing with the toy. In other words, the elbow, forearm, and wrist must work properly or hand and finger coordination will be compromised.

Upper-extremity casting can position those joints into correct alignment so that the muscles work more efficiently. The cast provides a slow, gradual stretch to the tight or contracted muscles, improving the range of movement while maintaining correct alignment. This can facilitate the child's ability to have better active reach and/or to provide the stability needed for functional activities that require prehension.

Therapists who use the Neuro-Developmental Treatment (NDT) approach recognize that this effective hands-on method does not exist in isolation and will include other treatment methods as needed to get the results they are seeking. Thus, although casting is not specifically an NDT component, therapists sometimes use this technique to achieve alignment, which is the basis for posture and movement.

Types of Casts

The most frequently used casts are the long arm cast, the rigid circular elbow cast, and the wrist cast.

Long arm cast

The long arm cast covers the entire surface of the arm from below the axilla (armpit) to the hand. It includes the elbow, forearm, and wrist. Tightness and spasticity in the forearm and elbow often cause a pronated forearm (palm facing

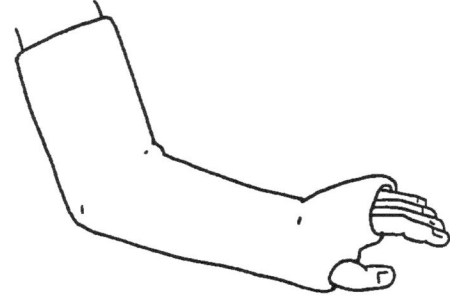

Figure 1a. Long arm cast, elbow flexed, forearm in pronation.

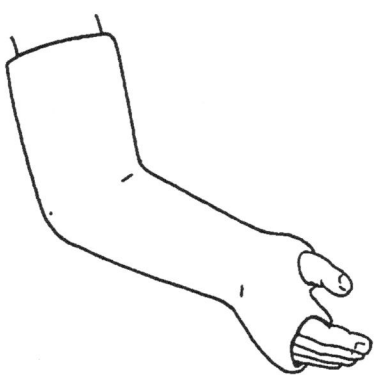

Figure 1b. Long arm cast, elbow more extended, forearm more supinated.

down) and a flexed elbow, which aligns the hand poorly for grasp. Initially, the cast might position the arm with the forearm in pronation and the elbow flexed (Figure 1a). A series of casts gradually positions the forearm into supination (palm facing up) while also lengthening the elbow into extension (Figure 1b). This puts the arm in better alignment during strengthening activities of the shoulder-girdle muscles. The shoulder joints are important because they place the elbow and forearm in position for reach and grasp.

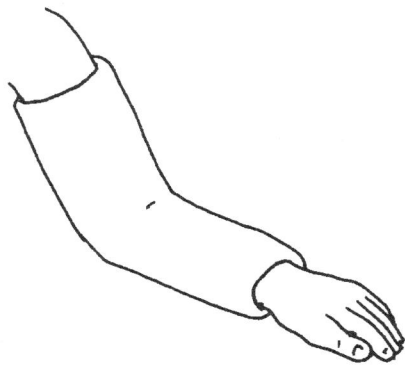

Figure 2. Rigid circular elbow cast.

Rigid circular elbow cast

The rigid circular elbow cast extends from the axilla to the wrist. When spasticity pulls the arm into elbow flexion, straightening the arm for reaching is difficult. An elbow cast can lengthen the elbow flexors gradually (Figure 2) and rebalance the elbow extensors. This cast is helpful while the child practices reaching in various planes to strengthen the tricep muscles and assists by gradually positioning the elbow into extension for weight bearing.

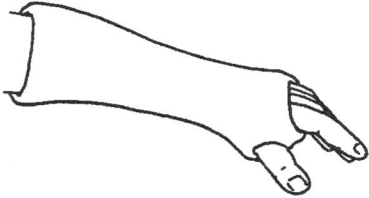

Figure 3. Wrist cast.

Wrist cast

The wrist cast provides stability and improved range at the wrist joint for a child with poor wrist and finger movements (Figure 3). The cast can hold the wrist in a variety of positions, depending on the limitation of range at the wrist joint and the increased spasticity. Serial casting can increase range of motion at the wrist gradually, to facilitate finger movement for grasp, pinch, and prehension while wearing the cast. Additionally, the cast can improve alignment to facilitate skin care as well as prepare for wearing a follow-up maintenance splint.

Cast Management

Cast manufacturers use plaster, which is somewhat heavy, or synthetic materials, which are lighter in weight. Regardless of the type of cast applied, it is important that you help your child manage the cast. Make sure that the cast dries thoroughly and remains properly molded. Generally it takes 48 hours for the plaster cast to become completely dry. Inspect the skin near the cast edges daily, and check the arm or hand for signs of swelling, coldness, or numbness. The child initially might complain of discomfort, but this might be due to the constant gentle stretch. After the first or second day, the arm should become more relaxed while in the cast.

Avoid getting the cast wet. Take special care to wrap the cast with a plastic bag during bathing. If the cast becomes wet, it tends to soften and becomes ineffective. Don't scratch the skin under the cast.

Goals

Casting goals vary, depending on the severity of the child's arm. Because the child is an active participant while the cast is on, it is vital to encourage movement of specific muscles depending on the type of cast applied. Movement with alignment while wearing a cast can improve shoulder-girdle stability and also might assist with strengthening weak muscles to facilitate better arm placement for prehension. This can happen during active arm placement and hand function with daily self-care tasks or play activities.

Goals of upper-extremity casting include one or more of the following:

- improve range for function
- improve range for hygiene
- improve range to fit a definitive splint
- lengthen muscles and rebalance muscle actions
- improve active reach
- improve prehension

Developing proximal stability for distal mobility is a basic NDT principle. The arm and hand can work more efficiently and with more control if the dynamic movements are working off of a stable base of support. The cast provides that support. Examples of activities based on that principle are upper-extremity dressing while wearing the long arm or elbow cast, and lower-extremity dressing while wearing the wrist cast.

For upper-extremity dressing while wearing the long arm or elbow cast, encourage active movement. Although your child will be unable to flex or extend the elbow, rotate the forearm, or use full wrist movement, you can encourage general gross-arm placement. Actively lifting the casted arm overhead will improve shoulder-girdle stability and strength. Provide a chair that supports your child so that it is easier for him or her to sit well balanced. Have your child use the uninvolved arm to place the casted arm in the sleeve hole of the T-shirt, shirt, or jacket. If donning a T-shirt, your child then will pull the T-shirt over the neck with the uninvolved arm, put the uninvolved arm through the sleeve, pull down the shirt, and adjust the front. If your child is unable to dress him- or herself, encourage him or her to lift the cast actively to push the arm through the sleeve hole.

For lower-extremity dressing while wearing the wrist cast, encourage active grasp with the casted hand while putting on or taking off pants, socks, or shoes. Provide a chair that supports your child so that it is easier for him or her to assume a sit-to-stand position. Try having the child who requires more assistance dress him- or herself while seated on the floor or sitting against a corner wall. Encourage bilateral hand grasp for pulling pants up or pushing them down. Encourage the child to use both hands during the various steps of dressing in underpants, socks, and shoes.

Summary

When the casting program is completed, it is important to continue to follow up with active movements with the muscles in the lengthened position. Help your child continue to develop the active arm, elbow, forearm, and hand movements needed for functional skills of daily self-care and play activities. Encourage symmetry and active grasp by asking your child for help with the laundry, moving clothes from the hamper to a basket, carrying the basket to the laundry room, sorting the clothes, and placing them in the washer and then in the dryer. Your child also can fold laundry, starting with washcloths, hand towels, and bath towels. Suggest carrying piles of folded laundry with both hands and placing them on shelves and in drawers.

Most importantly, have fun guiding your child through these new movements and watching new skills emerge!

For more clarification of Neuro-Developmental Treatment (NDT) theory and how it influences therapy for children, see Article 1.2 by Judith Bierman, titled "Philosophy, Theory, and Principles: The What, Why, and How of NDT."

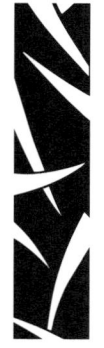

How Can I Get That Arm Straight? The Quest for Elbow Extension

Diane Berg McCormack, M.S., OTR

3.6

Occupational therapists continually encounter children with cerebral palsy who can't control their elbow movements. Parents complain of difficulty in dressing and undressing because of flexed (bent) elbows and fisted hands. The arm collapses when the child tries to side sit or crawl on hands and knees. Reaching for objects or catching a ball is impossible when the child's arm stays bent and tucked close to the body or up and back. Activities that are easy for most children are frustrating for the child who can't stabilize a bowl while eating or a sheet of paper while writing (Figure 1).

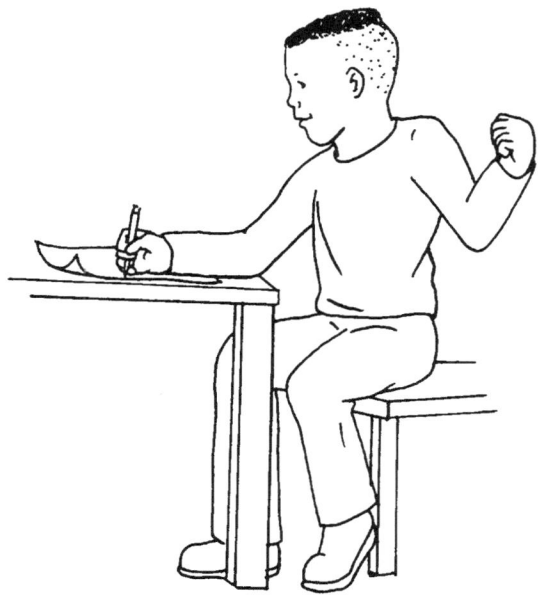

Figure 1.

What causes the elbow to be so difficult to control? Despite so much flexion and high muscle tone, the child with neuromotor disabilities has real weakness in the neck, shoulder, trunk, and hip muscles, resulting in postural instability. The child then tries to solve this problem by using immature movement patterns such as the high-guard position of one or both arms. Typically developing young infants use this high-guard position when they are beginning to roll, sit, stand, and walk to reinforce an upright trunk as they move, especially up against gravity (Figure 2).

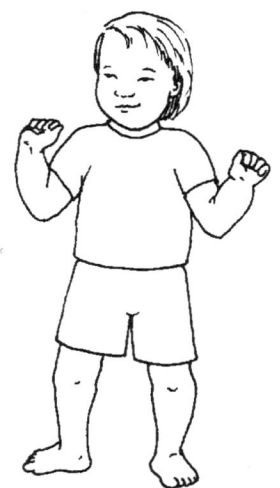

Figure 2.

The child with hemiplegia (one side of the body affected) sometimes holds in high guard with one arm in order to move or reach with the other arm. The child with quadriplegia (total body affected) might hold with both arms in order to remain upright in sitting or standing. Unfortunately, these static arm positions interfere with the development of more dynamic trunk and arm movements. The high-guard pattern reinforces muscle stiffness and limits specific muscles that straighten the elbow, turn the palm up, straighten the wrist, and extend the fingers and thumb.

During direct treatment, therapists usually focus on Neuro-Developmental Treatment (NDT) techniques such as:

- neuromuscular facilitation (helping the child use muscles appropriately)
- inhibition (preventing the child from using nonproductive movements)
- proper alignment (lining up joints so that they work efficiently)

What can parents and other caregivers do to reinforce the therapy goals of muscle strengthening and facilitation of more mature dynamic movements? How can they incorporate these activities into functional, age-appropriate occupational tasks such as self-help, play, and school work?

One method that has worked for many children is the use of a soft, reinforced elbow splint, constructed from neoprene or heavy cloth. It can assist the child in a variety of ways during therapy as well as daily living activities throughout the day. With a parent's help, a therapist can custom-measure the splint, and they can construct it together. A commercial company can fabricate the splint if construction is too time consuming.

Funding

The child's therapist can request a physician's order for soft reinforced elbow splints. A local equipment dealer then can bill private insurance or government medical assistance for the splints. If no other funding source is available, parents might wish to pay privately for splints because they tend to be reasonably priced.

Purpose of the Splint

The soft reinforced elbow splint has many purposes:

- to help straighten the elbow, using the elbow splint.
- to promote weight bearing on a straight arm in a variety of positions (side sitting [Figure 3], all fours, and standing) and during transitional movement patterns (moving from side sit to all fours and back to side sit).
- to hold the affected arm in a straightened position during two-hand activities to perform bilateral functional tasks, such as eating, paper/pencil tasks, and catching a large ball.
- to facilitate grasp on tricycle handlebars by custom modification to the elbow angle (Figure 4).

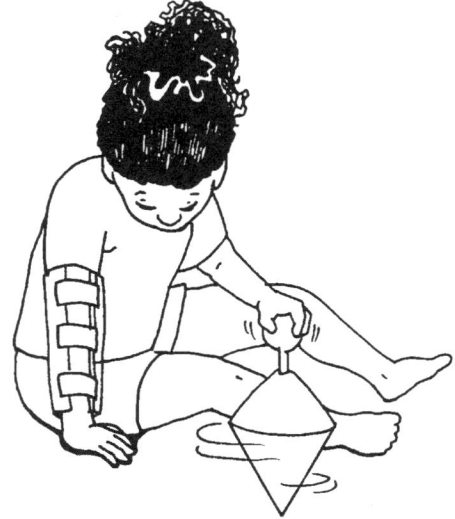

Figure 3.

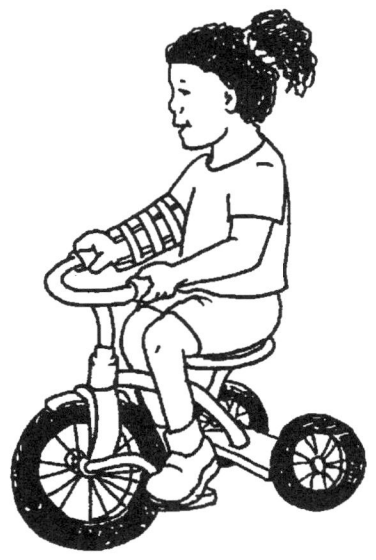

Figure 4.

Splint Pattern

To make a splint, you'll need neoprene or heavy cloth (such as denim), metal stays or splinting material, three or four 1-inch D-rings, and 3/4-inch to 1-inch wide Velcro® strips (6–8 inches of both hook and pile sides, 3 inches of hook side only; see Figure 5 and the sources listed at the end of this article). Start by making a pattern on paper. Remember that the goal of the splint is to prevent elbow flexion by covering the majority of the arm, but the splint shouldn't cut off circulation in the armpit or interfere with wrist extension during weight bearing.

Measure around the child's upper arm (1–2 inches below the armpit) and the child's forearm (1–2 inches above the wrist). Then add 2–3 inches for growth and clothing. Next, measure the length of your child's arm from 1–2 inches below the armpit to 1–2 inches above the wrist. Transfer these measurements to a paper pattern, slightly curving the upper and lower edges of the pattern to accommodate the narrowing at the lower edge. (Note: If your child is going to wear a hand or forearm wrist splint in addition to the elbow splint, you might need to modify the width and length to accommodate the other splint.)

Determine how many stays you'll need. Stays run along the length of the arm to hold the arm straight and prevent the elbow from bending. The stays usually are straight or manufactured to a specific angle required for a task. A very small arm might require only one or two stays. Most children need three stays. A very large, strong, or older child might need four stays. You can make the stays of metal or have them custom made from durable splinting material.

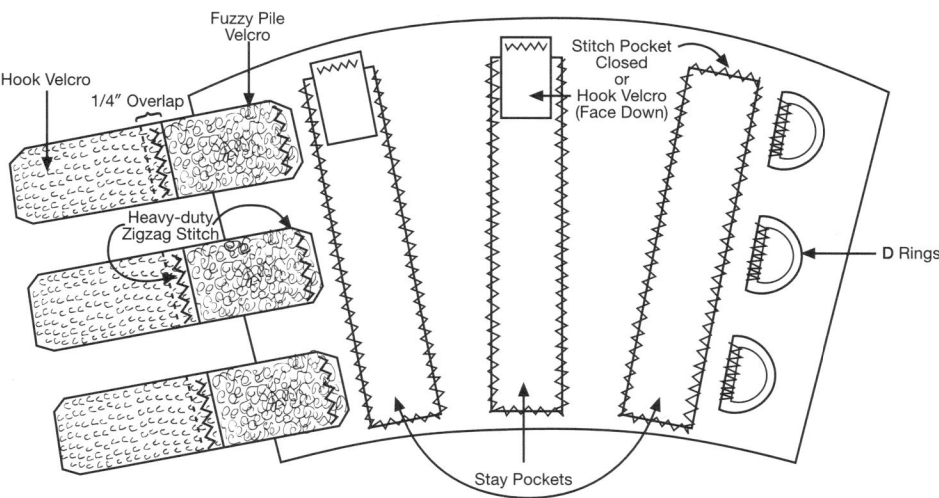

Figure 5.

Cut the neoprene or denim according to the paper pattern you've made, and fit it around your child's arm to make sure it fits with adequate overlap. Cut strips of neoprene or fabric about 1/2-inch wider and longer than the splint stays. Space these stay pockets around the splint (being careful not to place a stay in the area of overlap at either end of the splint). Use a wide zigzag to stitch the sides and one end of each strip to the body of the splint. Insert a stay into each long pocket, then stitch the ends of the long pockets closed, or stitch a small strip of hook Velcro® on the body of the splint just above the upper, open end of each pocket. The Velcro hooks will grab onto the fabric if it's at all fuzzy and effectively seal the pocket, keeping the stay in place yet allowing you to remove the stays to bend or straighten them as needed or to wash the splint.

Using heavy-duty thread, stitch three or four D-rings directly onto the splint fabric next to the outermost stay on one end of the splint. (For a left-arm splint, place D-rings on the right end of the splint; for a right-arm splint, stitch the rings on the left end.)

Cut three or four 2-inch lengths of Velcro (as many lengths as D-rings on the splint). Peel the two layers apart and lay the strips end-to-end with hooks and fuzzy pile facing up. Overlap the ends of the strips 1/4 inch and stitch them together securely. This makes a 3 3/4-inch strip of Velcro with hooks on one end and fuzzy pile on the other. Complete this step for the other strips of Velcro.

Position the Velcro strips on the other end of the splint opposite the D-rings, with the hooks and fuzzy pile facing up. Place about 1 inch of the fuzzy end of the strip onto the splint. Stitch through the Velcro and the splint fabric securely, letting the rest of the length of the strip extend from the edge of the splint.

To place the splint on the child's arm, wrap the splint around the arm (D-rings, stay pockets, and Velcro strips on the outside), insert the strips through the D-rings, then fasten the strips back on themselves.

Summary

A soft reinforced elbow splint can help the child perform everyday functional tasks while generating more mature movement patterns in the shoulder girdle, arm, and hand.

Resources

Neoprene

Special Products for Special Kids
Benik Corporation
11871 Silverdale Way NW, Suite #107
Silverdale, Washington 98383
800-442-8910

Fabric

The Medi-Kid Co.
P.O. Box 5398
Hemet, CA 92544
888-463-3543

For more clarification of Neuro-Developmental Treatment (NDT) theory and how it influences therapy for children, see Article 1.2 by Judith Bierman, titled "Philosophy, Theory, and Principles: The What, Why, and How of NDT."

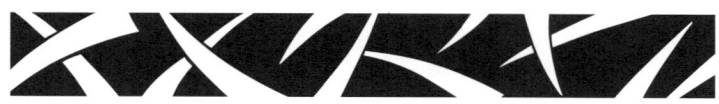

Section 4

Movement and Touch

Learning to Move

Gloria Frolek Clark, M.S., OTR/L, FAOTA

Learning to move is a critical part of a child's development. Whether it's moving the whole body across the floor toward a parent or moving an arm to reach for a toy, movement offers challenge and fosters independence.

What drives children to move? Key influences are their curiosity to explore the environment and their motivation to obtain objects or seek people. Yet, movement sometimes requires extreme effort. Think about any child pulling to stand for the first time. After several unintended plops on the floor, the child continues to try! We watch the typically developing child struggle over and over to learn a task and realize how important mastery of movement is to that child.

Parents of children with cerebral palsy or with developmental delay watch their children struggle for much longer periods of time to overcome gravity and to move through space. Some parents are anxious to have their child move; others are worried that movement will mean increased danger, and they have mixed feelings about their child learning to move independently.

Although most children learn to move on their own, some children must be taught. The innate desire to move motivates many to use any method to achieve this goal. Other children try for a while and then give up. When certain children require extra time to organize their actions and carry them out, the people around them usually think they are unable to do the task. Anxious to help, they might perform the tasks themselves rather than allowing the children enough time to make an attempt. The children thus receive the message that if they wait long enough, someone will do it for them. The following example illustrates the importance of waiting.

A 4-year-old girl with profound mental and physical disabilities attended an early childhood special education preschool. She had demonstrated the ability to blink her eyes if the lights were too bright and to moan if she wanted attention. Although she sometimes moved her head slightly to the left, no one was sure if this movement was voluntary because they hadn't observed any voluntary head movements. The teacher and occupational therapist wanted to teach the child to use a microswitch so that she could interact with her environment. No one was sure if she could learn to turn it on. By recording the amount of time it took for her to turn her head after being cued, they discovered that she consistently required about 90 seconds to organize her movements and make a response! No one had ever waited that long for her. As people began waiting, she began to increase her movements and, over time, decreased her response time to 40 seconds! She also began to smile and explore her environment by turning her head toward sounds and people.

The sensory information children receive during movement provides critical new knowledge to the central nervous system—information the child can use when planning new movements. When children have a limited repertoire of strategies, their actions can be limited as well. For example, a child who has learned to roll will have to change direction when an object blocks the movement. Learning to turn the body provides the nervous system with new information it can use in the future. The child's increased ability to problem solve results in enhanced planning and motor performance.

The development of movement occurs in a systematic manner, with control of the head usually present before control of the arms and legs. However, as parents know, children with movement disorders sometimes develop at a different rate or sequence. Goals will depend upon the age and specific limitations of the child.

The purpose of this article is not to discuss the development of movement. Instead, the goal is to focus on how parents and caregivers of children with cerebral palsy and other movement disorders can motivate their children to learn to move. Learning is an active, not passive, process. Children will learn if they are motivated to try and allowed the freedom to explore. Parents play a critical role in both of these aspects.

Cognition, vision, and hearing are important areas that parents also must consider when attempting to motivate a child to learn. You might find that modifications are necessary for children with sensory loss and children with low cognitive skills who sometimes require more assistance and different activities to motivate them.

Neuro-Developmental Treatment (NDT) Principles

NDT principles are the basis for these strategies.

- **NDT Principle:** Knowledge of children's current voluntary movement strategies is necessary for parents and therapists to plan treatment.

Learning to Move

Activity: Improving your observation skills

Method: Keep a notebook, listing all the movements your child can make voluntarily. You might want to set up categories such as hand, leg, and body movements. Your child might be able to do some activities without your help, whereas other emerging skills require more practice. Consider putting a star by the skills that are emerging, because those will be the easiest for you to help your child develop. Next, list objects or people who seem to motivate your child. Continue to add to this list as your child masters new skills. You probably will find that in a week or two you are much more aware of these actions and motivators, and can share this wealth of knowledge with the professionals working with your child. This activity also is important because it helps you rediscover all that your child can do at this point in time and serves as an ongoing list of accomplishments.

If your child has few active movements, list any part of the movement that occurs. By paying attention, many families have begun to notice these partial movements. For example, one family noticed that their child's eyes turned toward the phone when it rang. Another parent noticed that the child rolled toward the door when the garage door opened, which showed that, although the child could not move physically in that direction, he still was able to connect where the sound came from and what would happen next (cause and effect).

- **NDT Principle:** Parents can assist their children to move, through special handling—a way of using the hands to add sensory input.

  Activity: Consider ways to encourage your child's movements throughout daily routines.

  Method: Helping your child feel the correct way of moving is important input to the central nervous system. Performing the activity during a naturally occurring time also helps establish a link to that activity. For example, if your child is able to sit alone in the middle of the floor but can't get into or out of sitting, you could begin teaching that skill. Instead of simply picking your child up from the floor, help move both hands to the floor on one side of the body, slowly getting into a side-lying position, in preparation for your lifting (Figure 1).

  In a similar way, place your child in side lying and help him or her to push up to sitting with both hands. Doing this throughout the day provides the correct feeling of movement and many opportunities for learning to move. It is critical that you decrease assistance as your child begins to participate in the activity, so as to reduce your child's dependence.

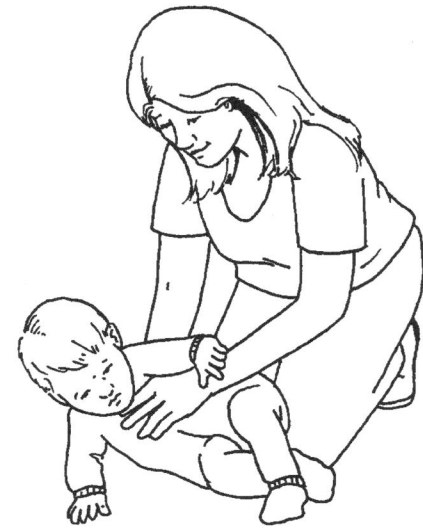

Figure 1.

- **NDT Principle:** Children learn about their bodies and environment through self-directed movements.

  Activity: Encourage active exploration.

  Method: Using the motivators you've already identified, foster your child's desire to move and explore. For example:

  – Encourage your child to roll or crawl toward you (whole-body movements). Start close to your child, then increase the distance as your child's skills improve and safe navigation around the house increases. Mealtime can motivate a child to learn how to get out of sitting and roll toward the kitchen as you stand there and call. Placing or hanging toys in various parts of a room also might increase your child's motivation to explore. Use toys with sounds if your child has visual problems. Sensory exploration is important for learning about size, textures, and sounds. Crawling over various surfaces, under tables, and into small spaces helps children learn about the size and shape of their own bodies in relation to other objects. These activities are especially motivating for young children.

  – Place objects near the child's hand and wait for a response (arm and hand movements). Touch the child's palm with objects you know are motivating because of their color, sound, or texture. Because children love to explore kitchen cupboards and drawers, keep safe and fun objects such as pots (with covers), muffin tins, and plastic storage containers in an area designated for them. Sensori-motor activities can include toys with a variety of textures, water toys, and objects hidden in a pan of rice. Children also love Mylar™ wrapping paper because it crinkles and doesn't tear easily.

- **NDT Principle:** Children refine movement patterns based on experience (sensory-motor-sensory feedback).

  Activity: Provide opportunities for children to problem solve new movement strategies.

  Method: As your child gains more independence in performing a skill, it is important to provide additional opportunities for learning. For example, if your child has learned to push up on extended arms from the stomach position on the floor, what will happen on a soft surface such as the bed? Sometimes you might need to set up barriers such as pillows and cushions to challenge your child to learn to move around them. Or, when a child has learned to use a certain spoon, provide one with a different shape and watch how the spoon-to-mouth movement changes. These challenges help the child grow cognitively as well as motorically. Being able to figure out how to move is critical. Many children are stuck in a few positions because they don't know how to move their bodies in new ways.

Precautions

As your child learns to move and explore, it is necessary to look more carefully at the safety of your home. People have found that getting down on the floor at the child's level presents an interesting view of hazards that weren't otherwise visible!

Use caution in any activity that you think could be harmful to your child. For example, if your child has low muscle tone (weakness), pulling on his or her arm during some of these assistive movements could result in subluxation (joint coming out of the socket). Talk with your child's therapist or physician if you have any questions about specific handling techniques.

Summary

Exploratory movement in the world is critical to child development. But learning to move can be hard work! Sometimes children give up trying because it takes them so long to plan and perform the movement that someone else is willing to do for them.

Parents have an important role in finding fun and motivating activities that will help their children learn to move, explore objects, and interact with people in their environment. You can encourage your child by providing many opportunities to practice new skills.

For more clarification of Neuro-Developmental Treatment (NDT) theory and how it influences therapy for children, see Article 1.2 by Judith Bierman, titled "Philosophy, Theory, and Principles: The What, Why, and How of NDT."

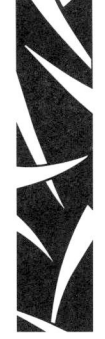

Practicing Basic Transitions: Foundations for All Movement Skills

Vickie Meade, M.P.H., PT

The world of the infant is in his or her parents' arms. Your child spends many hours every day being lifted and carried by you, and played with while sitting in your lap or on the couch or floor next to you. This world of your arms and lap can be an effective starting place for teaching something very important to your infant or young child who continues to wish to be close to you—movement skills.

An infant who has had a difficult start in his or her development might not be as comfortable holding the body upright against the force of gravity. The trunk muscles might seem weaker (floppy), and the arms and legs sometimes stiffen in response to being held. If a child learns only how to position the arms and legs to hold him- or herself stable against gravity, the balance muscles of the trunk don't get a chance to develop strength. In addition, the child will use arm and leg muscles to keep the body in the sagittal (forward and backward) plane of movement. However, to be successful holding and balancing against gravity, your child must learn to be comfortable with experiencing and moving in a lateral plane (sideward).

How do we help your baby learn appropriate movement skills? Therapists using the Neuro-Developmental Treatment (NDT) approach traditionally have followed developmental sequences in treatment planning. For example, if a child could not lift his or her head when lying on the stomach, gaining control of the head in prone would be the first goal addressed rather than working in a sitting or side-lying position. Although therapists use their knowledge and understanding of normal development to help them with their observation skills, current research provides new information about how individuals learn and control movement. Therefore, therapists consider many additional factors, particularly kinesiology and mechanics of movement, when planning treatment.

Sagittal and Lateral Planes of Movement

It is important to understand the difference between sagittal and lateral planes of movement (Figure 1). Infants and young children with weaker trunk muscles easily learn to use their stronger back muscles (in the upper parts of their bodies) and their stronger hip muscles and behind-knee muscles (in the lower part of their bodies) to help hold themselves stable against gravity. They use these muscles to hold still in certain positions and to move backward and forward. Place yourself in sitting, and rock backward and forward. You use hip and knee muscles to help you bend forward and upper back muscles to help you move backward. These muscles keep you balanced without a lot of effort. This is movement in the sagittal (forward-backward) plane.

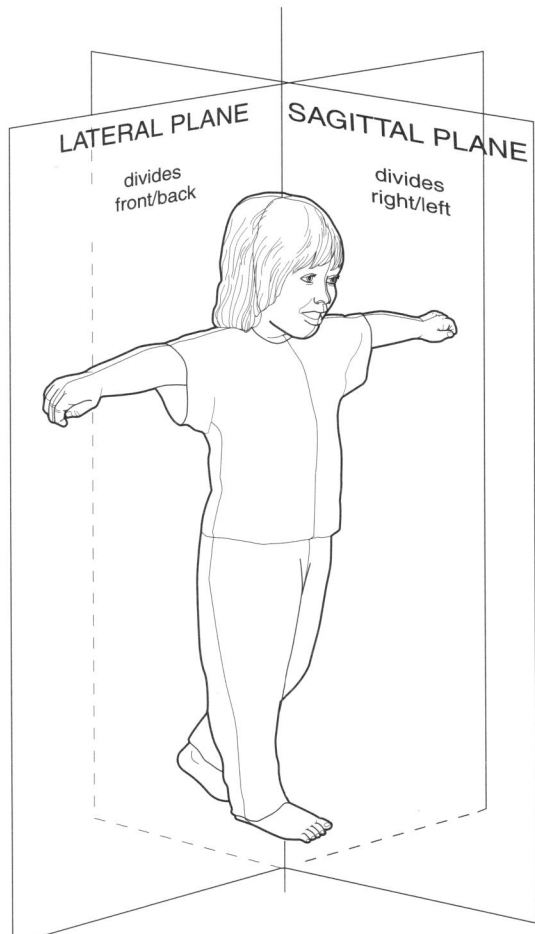

Figure 1. Planes of the body.

Now, in sitting again, move from side to side. You will notice that your head tilts one way and your body or trunk curves so that you do not fall over. This is movement in the lateral (side-to-side) plane. It requires more muscle work of the trunk, more effort, and, most importantly, balance.

Now try this side-to-side movement while keeping your head and body very straight. Sit toward one side and notice how this becomes harder. If sideward movement causes

Practicing Basic Transitions: Foundations for All Movement Skills

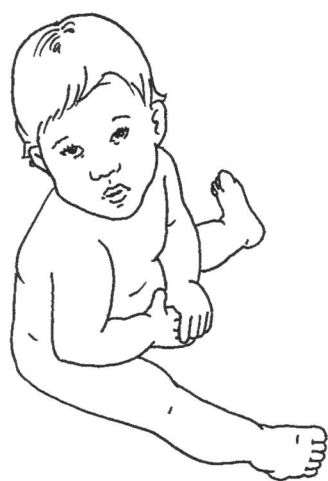

Figure 2. Sitting and moving in the lateral plane.

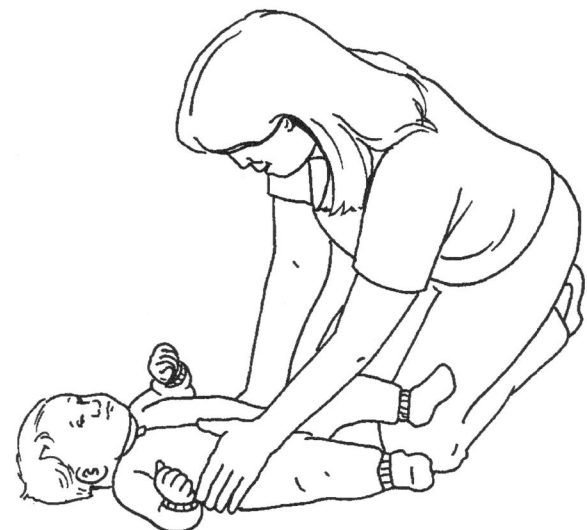

Figure 3. Side-lying lift: Hold in center of body.

your child to fall over, he or she will make every effort to try not to go sideward! The child might move the legs wide apart so that the head and trunk are able to move only forward and backward (Figure 2). Because movement in the lateral plane is harder to control, your child will need your help to develop it. (Movement in the forward-backward sagittal plane will develop with or without your help.) Movement side-to-side in the lateral plane is important because it helps prepare for balance in crawling and walking by assisting development of the muscles around the shoulder, trunk, and hips.

Development of Control in the Lateral Plane

How does control in this lateral plane usually develop, and how can you help your child learn this control? Infants first experience lateral movement when rolling. The first roll often is accidental. The child pushes up on straight arms, loses balance sideward, and falls over to the back. This often is a surprise to the child, who then will experiment with this new movement by pushing up again, taking just enough weight on one arm and adjusting the head and trunk toward the opposite side in order to stay balanced in the tummy position. The child who doesn't like to be on the tummy won't experiment with pushing up high enough on the arms to be in a position to fall over, and thus, won't have the opportunity to experiment with balance in this position. Try to place your child on his or her stomach often.

Side-lying lift

To help your child experience this lateral movement, you can roll him to the side each time you lift him up to carry him (Figures 3, 4, and 5). This experience in side lying will give him an opportunity to practice lifting his head and

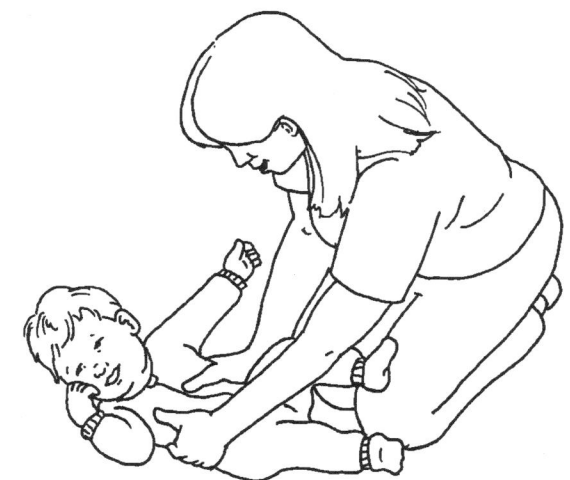

Figure 4. Side-lying lift: Roll onto side.

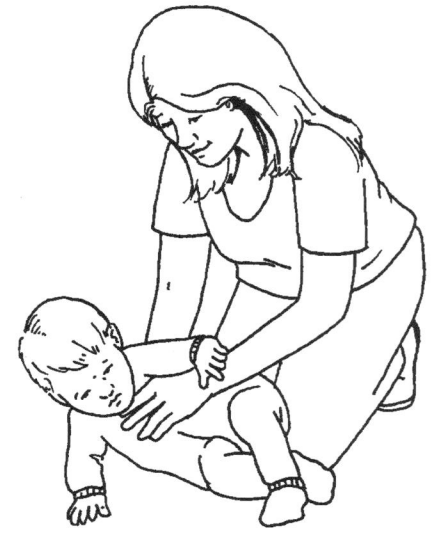

Figure 5. Side-lying lift: Lift in air while child is on side.

Practicing Basic Transitions: Foundations for All Movement Skills

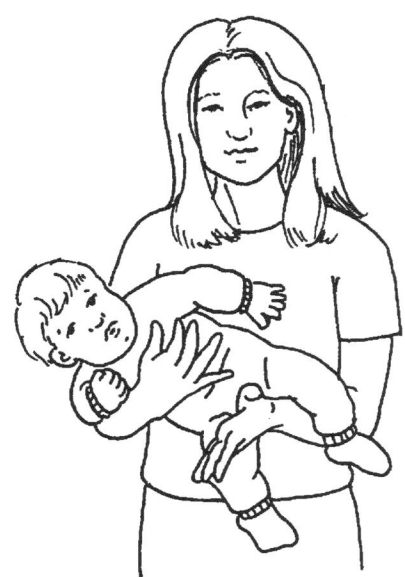

Figure 6. Side-lying carry position.

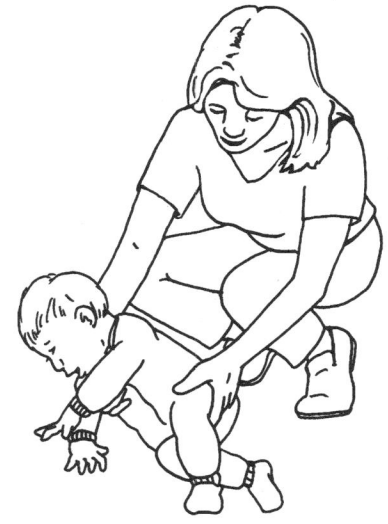

Figure 7. Setdown.

body sideward as you start to move him into space. These are the same head and trunk movements that a child without disabilities would be practicing in order to stay balanced on the tummy. Now you can carry your child in this side-lying position (Figure 6).

Side-lying carry

Your child also can experience these head and trunk movements in the lateral plane by the way that you hold him and carry him around. Hold the child on his side with his back against your chest, first toward your right side. Place your right arm under his shoulder and your left arm between his legs. Tilt him so that you feel him want to move his head sideward as he tries to move his head and body into a straighter position against you. Again, the child is using these head and trunk movements to balance and adjust his body against gravity, using the supportive base of your body and arms. Try to give only enough support so that he can do most of it himself and still be successful. Be sure to try this also on the opposite side.

Side-lying setdown

The third component of this series of movements is called the setdown, which is the reverse of the lift. Hold your child again on his side while placing him slowly back down on the floor. As you near the floor, allow time for the child to adjust to this new position. Watch and wait to see if he will move one arm out or tilt his head and body away from the floor. As the child comes in contact with the floor, lower him slowly so that he can choose either to roll to the tummy or to the back from this side-lying position (Figure 7).

From side lying to side sitting and more

Advance this entire series in stages as your child becomes stronger in adjusting the head and body, and anticipates and becomes familiar with the routine. Eventually, you will be able to lift your child up to a side sit, carry in side sit, and set down in side-sit positions. This allows the child's shoulders to become strong and stable. The shoulder muscles will help support the head and ribs and allow the muscles around the lower trunk to work effectively. You also can advance this series of lifts, carries, and setdowns to include the all-fours and standing positions as the child adjusts to being higher up against gravity.

The side-lying lift, carry, and setdown series forms a basis for a routine of movements you can practice first by going through the day, step by step. Start by mimicking wake-up time in the morning. Go to your child's crib and lift by rolling her to the side. Move her into the carry position and set her down on her side on the changing table, bed, or floor, wherever you usually change and dress her.

After dressing, roll your child to the side and lift and carry her into the kitchen for breakfast. Place your child into her chair. (As your child gains more skill, you can modify this setdown into the chair.) Then lift her out of the chair, move into a side-lying carry, and go into the living room to place her on the floor in a side-lying position for play. Depending on her skill level, you can leave your child on her side with towel rolls behind her or place her more toward her tummy with a towel roll in front. You also could place her on a firm pillow or wedge to have her body in side lying, but more at an angle so that she can see more easily (and practice lifting her head sideward). Adjust this position often, depending on the child's play interests and movement skill/tolerance in side lying. The eventual goal, of course, is to incorporate these routines into everyday life.

Summary

Routines form the basis for children to experience and learn about movement. They learn what their bodies are able to do, the limits of their bodies in relationship to the world, and choices about movements that they are able to make even when they have very few movements of their own.

The lift, carry, and setdown routine is the basic building block of movement routines and can help your child develop stability by increasing control of movement in the lateral plane. Movement in the lateral plane prepares the neck, shoulder, and trunk muscles for work in balancing the body against gravity. Balance of the body against gravity allows for more movement options, choices, and experimentation. You are the primary vehicle for your child to experience this movement control through the world of your arms.

Figure 1 adapted and reprinted with permission from *Spatial, Temporal, and Physical Analysis of Motor Control* by Diane Berg McCormack and Kathy Riske Perrin, published by Therapy Skill Builders, a division of The Psychological Corporation, 1-800-228-0752, ISBN 0761643788.

For more clarification of Neuro-Developmental Treatment (NDT) theory and how it influences therapy for children, see Article 1.2 by Judith Bierman, titled "Philosophy, Theory, and Principles: The What, Why, and How of NDT."

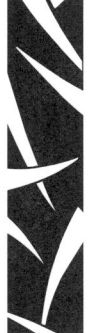

A Positive Perspective on Atypical Development: Understanding Why Your Child Moves This Way

Suzanne M. Davis, RPT

Historically, atypical development has been described as being *abnormal* and dictated by the brain. However, the more therapists learn from observing children and from research, the more we understand why children with neurological impairment and developmental delays move the way they do, and what we can do to help them reach their potential. Recent research tells us that children are moving in the best way that they can at a certain moment in time, given all the possibilities and all the limitations of their bodies. Sometimes it is truly incredible to see how creative children are as they figure out how to move and function despite their disabilities.

The strategies that these children use often are very similar to strategies that the typical baby uses before she has full active control of her body. For example, when a typical baby is lying on her tummy and tries to push her body up before she has adequate muscle activity in her lower spine and hips, she will use the hamstring muscles (in the back of the thigh) to help. When she gets older, her spine and hip muscles will be strong enough so that she doesn't need the hamstrings. Many older children with disabilities continue to use the hamstrings the same way for the same reason.

Postural or stabilizer muscles help hold our bodies upright against gravity and help us keep our balance. A baby or child who has an injury to the brain has weakened postural muscles. The child still wants to get up and function in his world. In order to do this, he will use muscles that have not weakened, usually those that move the arms and legs, called mobilizer muscles. You might already have noticed that your child's trunk feels weak and floppy but his arms, his legs, and sometimes his neck might feel stiff.

The child is using the mobilizer muscles instead of the stabilizer muscles to help support the body in upright postures. Unfortunately, some of the consequences of this strategy are that the child now is limited in the use of her arms for reaching, her eyes for exploring, and her legs for moving. Another consequence can be a tightening of the muscles. The more the child practices holding her body this way, the stronger a habit it becomes.

Did you know that typical babies are born with some muscles that are tight? Remember that the typical baby is curled up in the fetal position when he is born. When he lies on his tummy, the fetal position places a lot of weight and deep pressure on the upper chest. This actually helps lengthen the upper chest muscles. Babies who are atypical and those who are premature are weak and won't have this curled-up position, so they'll miss the opportunity to lengthen these upper chest muscles (often referred to as the pecs.)

Another area of tightness in the typical newborn is at the front of the hips. As the baby lifts her head and pushes up higher by pushing through her arms, she gently stretches out the tight hip muscles (hip flexors). This process takes about 6 months. The child with a neurological impairment doesn't always learn how to push up through the arms. Remember that the arms are busy helping to support posture. The baby's shoulders might be elevated to support the head, and the arms might be tucked against her sides. If the child doesn't push up, then she won't be able to stretch out her muscles. The muscle tightness persists, and this drastically changes how the child learns to move her body. When postural muscles are weak and other muscles are tight, the number of options the child has for movement are limited.

As an experiment, sit in a chair at a table with your feet planted on the floor, place your arms on the table, and lean some of your weight on your arms. Now keep your trunk in the same position and lift your arms up off the table. Pay attention to the muscles in your hips. Did you feel your hip muscles get active? These are the postural muscles that stabilize your hips. Now repeat the experiment again, only this time pretend that your hip muscles don't work. Do your best to turn them off and now try to lift your arms up. Cheat any way you can! It's very difficult, isn't it? Some creative ways of cheating are pulling your head and neck way back, leaning over on one arm to free up the other, leaning into the table so your chest rests there, or putting your head down to lift the arms.

You have just experienced a tiny bit of what it might be like if your postural muscles didn't work. These strategies probably look familiar to you, because they are strategies that many children with neurological impairments use. In other words, they move that way not because of the brain injury itself, but because it makes sense to try these other strategies when one's postural muscles are weak.

As therapists, our overall goal is to improve function and make it more efficient. We want to help our children increase their options for functional movement. In order to do this, therapists will work to build on the children's strengths and the positive components of movement they do have. Therapists also will work to decrease the limitations (muscle tightness, increased or decreased stiffness, poor strength, etc.) and increase the variety of movement patterns children can use actively for successful function in the world.

However, there is much that families can do to help meet this basic goal of improving function. Every family spends a great deal of time with their child. Parents truly are the people who know their child the best. You have many opportunities to help your child achieve higher and more energy-efficient function, especially by understanding and using some of the principles of Neuro-Developmental Treatment (NDT), which follow guidelines derived from the current study of motor control:

- Obtain optimal alignment for movement efficiency in specific functional tasks.
- Progress the child toward energy-efficient work.
- Strengthen weak muscles within functional movement patterns.

An understanding of these principles is important if you want to use the following NDT handling techniques with your child at home.

- **Problem:** Some children sit with the pelvis tipped back and the spine rounded. This can result from weak postural muscles and tight or stiff hips. When the hips are stiff or the postural muscles are weak, the spine bends instead of the hips.

  Activity: Place your hand on the child's pelvis and gently bring it forward. Don't push if it feels tight. If you feel resistance, gently rock the pelvis from side to side. This helps tight muscles relax and can activate postural muscles. Slowly bring the pelvis into a perpendicular position (straight up). When you get the right alignment, the child will become more active, using and strengthening the postural muscles to hold the position independently.

- **Problem:** When some children begin to climb up into bed, on the couch, or into the car, they often are out of alignment and have a lot of difficulty. The climbing knee might be out to the side or crossed in front of the body instead of being directly under the hip.

  Activity: As the child begins to climb, help bring the hip directly over the knee. Putting the leg and the body in the right alignment enables the child to use muscles effectively, and using the muscles strengthens them. The child then will be able to push up onto the surface.

- **Problem:** Some children aren't strong enough yet to support the body in upright positions. The postural muscles are at risk of getting overstretched when the children collapse (and they do!).

  Activity: It is very important to support these children until they get stronger. Ask your therapist about various pieces of supportive equipment for sitting and standing. When you hold or carry your child, make sure that the spine is in a gentle, straight position with the bend at the hips, not in the back.

- **Problem:** When some children try to lift themselves up from the tummy, they can't lift the head very high. The bottom might lift up off the surface or the legs might get very stiff.

  Activity: You can help shift some of the body weight backward. Place your hand gently down on the child's bottom. Use only as much pressure as you would on a cotton ball. Give gentle pressure down toward the floor and slightly toward the feet. This makes it easier for the child to lift the head up and push with the arms.

When we, as parents and therapists, use a positive perspective to look at our children, we can understand better the reasons why they move the way they do. We can learn how to help them change their movements to achieve better function. If we really believe that our children have potential, we will do everything we can to help them reach that potential.

For more clarification of Neuro-Developmental Treatment (NDT) theory and how it influences therapy for children, see Article 1.2 by Judith Bierman, titled "Philosophy, Theory, and Principles: The What, Why, and How of NDT."

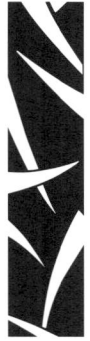

Minimizing the Problem of Learned Helplessness: What Can Parents Do to Help?

Kristen Birkmeier, M.S., PT

Learned helplessness is a term that means certain children have learned to depend on their parents or caregivers because it is more comforting and rewarding than achieving more and more activities independently. When children cannot and do not try to help when they are being dressed, fed, moved from one position to another, or objects are brought to them, parents essentially are caring for their every need.

All of us start out as tiny infants who are totally dependent upon adults for all our needs. But as babies, we learn to roll over, then move toward toys. We figure out how to get up into sitting and how to crawl on our hands and knees. Eventually, we learn to pull up to stand to reach things that are up off the floor, and finally, we learn to walk! As toddlers and preschoolers, we learn to eat, get dressed and undressed, take baths, ride tricycles, climb ladders, go down slides, run, and jump. We are getting ready for kindergarten.

But what happens if, as infants, we have difficulty learning to move and do things for ourselves? What if just holding the head up, rolling over, or sitting up without having to lean on our hands are skills that are very difficult for us to learn? If we needed someone else to help us all the time, how would we ever learn to take care of ourselves, play with other kids, go to school, and grow up and be on our own some day? What if life were just really hard? Wouldn't we grow up expecting our parents and others to do all the things that are too difficult for us to do? Wouldn't there always be someone there to take care of us and do anything we need, for our whole life? Would we really need to learn all those skills that would someday allow us to be self-sufficient?

You might be wondering what you can do to get started early in the process of expecting more independence from your child. Or if your child is presently very dependent, you might want very much to reverse this trend, especially if you believe that your child is capable of doing more for him- or herself.

How can you provide the support your child needs and, at the same time, communicate realistic expectations for independence? How can you help your child learn to move his or her own body, care for him- or herself, play and interact with people and objects in the environment, and get ready for formal education? What can you do to help your child begin to dream and work to realize those dreams? How can you maintain that delicate balance between providing the support and help your child needs, yet lead your child toward independence?

Time always is a major consideration, so you need to pick a time of day that allows you to place greater expectations on your child for actively participating in a movement or functional activity such as dressing, eating, bathing, and playing, and at the same time, doesn't create frustration and a time crunch for everyone.

Suggestions for an Infant

- When turning your baby from his tummy to his back or vice versa, start the movement from his bottom and see if he can bring his head and shoulders with the movement. When he is lying on his back, help him learn to bring his hands together in the air above his chest, to reach out for your face or objects that you hold out for him, and to hold objects and bring them up to his mouth.

- When picking up your baby, slowly help her get to sitting by lifting under both arms, then tipping her slowly to the left or right so she can work on holding up her head through the movement and eventually push up on one arm.

- When holding your baby on your lap, sometimes hold both sides of his trunk and seat him out away from you so that he can hold up his head. Then slowly tip him from side to side and forward/backward so that he can work to control his head against gravity. Hold objects out in front of him so that he can work to reach out and grasp the object. If reaching with one hand is easier than the other, encourage him to reach to the more difficult side, too.

- Make sure that your baby spends some time each day on her tummy so that she can learn to support on her arms, hold up her head to look around or talk to you, and work to develop the back muscles that are needed to roll over, push up onto her hands and knees, and get into sitting. Give her little nudges on one shoulder or the other so that she learns to shift her weight from side to side and reach out with either hand.

- With your baby sitting on your lap facing you, hold him on both sides of his trunk under his arms and help him to get up onto his feet, coming upward and toward you. Help him to bounce and stand on his legs with a little bend in his knees. This is something you can do with your baby from the time he is 4 or 5 months old.

Suggestions for a Toddler

- Always think about the different positions and activities that children the same age as your child are doing. Try to find ways to give your child an opportunity to participate in these age-appropriate activities and positions.

- If your child is 12 to 15 months old, help her pull up to stand through half-kneel at coffee tables or couches that are about the right height. Encourage play in standing as she supports her weight through her chest and arms on the furniture in front of her. Stimulate her to work on getting up and down, reaching down to a lower level that is higher than the floor level, etc. If your child is unable to walk, hold her trunk on both sides, tip her slightly forward, and encourage her to take steps to help walk across the room.

Suggestions for a Walker

- If your child is 18 to 24 months, add these activities: Help your child climb up and down stairs and furniture using his arms and legs. He will push up onto the higher level with his knees while pulling with his arms. Be sure that he turns onto his tummy to crawl down the stairs and alternates his legs, and ensure that he rolls on to his tummy before trying to get down from a couch or chair. Have your child help with dressing by pulling shirts off his head and pushing his arms through sleeves and his legs through pant legs.

- If your child is 2 to 3 years old, add these activities: Help your child move a riding toy and progress to a tricycle, even if you need to adapt it with special pedals and a trunk support for the seat in order for her to be able to sit upright.

Suggestions for a Preschooler or School-Age Child

- Explain to your child that you believe he can do more of the movement or activity than he has been doing, and that you want him to start doing more. Assure your child that you will help when the activity is too hard for him, but you really want him to try to do more of it for himself.

An important principle of Neuro-Developmental Treatment (NDT) involves teaching an infant, young child, or teenager how to be as independent as possible. Be sure to ask your physical therapist to work with you to teach your child how to change postural positions, move, and explore, and to help your child learn some method of moving independently to get where she needs or wants to go. At first, working against gravity is difficult, especially when your infant or young child is on her tummy, back, or hands and knees. Sometimes, the therapist will begin with your child in a more upright position such as sitting on a bench, standing, or moving between these postures. Because those more upright postures minimize the pull of gravity on your child's body, she can learn better head control, how to bear weight on her arms and legs, and how to use her trunk muscles more effectively for balance reactions. You can learn how to help your child gain control of her body in these postures so that she will be better able to get up off the floor to hands and knees, into sitting, up to kneeling, and eventually pull up onto the feet in standing independently or with minimal assistance.

Together, you and your therapist will begin to place appropriate expectations on your child so that he realizes early in the treatment process that you expect him to be actively involved in everyday activities as well as the therapy program. He will begin to realize that he can move about in his environment to explore and play and, at some point, learn to stand up onto his feet or out of his bed or wheelchair without your help, or with very little help. These are the building blocks your child needs in order to learn to care for himself independently some day.

You know best what your child can do and what you would like her to do to take a more active role. Start small, with small changes in your expectations, but start today. No matter how much you want to believe it, your child is not going to wake up some morning and magically be ready to participate more fully in the activities of daily life. You play the most important role in helping your child learn to take responsibility for her own body and developing some independence. You, your child, and your therapist can share ideas and suggestions. You all will be amazed at how quickly your child begins to make changes. It all starts with you setting different expectations for her! As you teach your child to move and take responsibility for her own body, she will begin to develop a positive self-image and build independence for now and in the future. Start today!

For more clarification of Neuro-Developmental Treatment (NDT) theory and how it influences therapy for children, see Article 1.2 by Judith Bierman, titled "Philosophy, Theory, and Principles: The What, Why, and How of NDT."

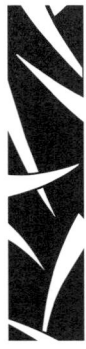

The Unique Physical Challenges of Children With Hypertonia

Marcia Stamer, PT

Children with hypertonia (increased muscle tone) represent the largest group of children with cerebral palsy. Sometimes they also have additional movement disorders such as athetosis and ataxia combined with their increased muscle tone.

These children usually are classified as quadriplegic (involvement of all four extremities, head, and trunk), diplegic (legs and eyes much more affected than arms and upper trunk), or hemiplegic (primarily on one side of the body). Many children do not fit neatly into these classifications, perhaps affected, for example, in legs, head, trunk, and only one arm. Or their diagnosis may change as they grow older and respond well to therapy, later being considered diplegic instead of quadriplegic.

Children who are affected very mildly can do most of what other children their age do, except for difficulties with skills such as running, writing, and pronouncing certain words. However, children who are very much affected cannot hold their heads up, use their arms to reach or grasp, or make more than a few sounds. Because of the wide range of abilities in children with hypertonia (and in all forms of cerebral palsy), we can't really paint a typical picture. However, some common characteristics are:

- Stiffness, in one or more parts of the body, that changes depending on the situation. The stiffness increases when the child gets excited, afraid, or angry, or when he tries very hard to do something new or difficult. The stiffness decreases and movement is easier when he feels confident about a particular skill. We often can help the child change the amount of this stiffness and how often it happens.

- Tendency to lose mobility, with joints developing contractures and muscles shortening, resulting in less range of motion. This develops over time as the muscles constantly contract rather than contracting and letting go. We can treat and minimize this problem, too, although not eliminate it.

- Using a limited number of muscles to make movements happen. For example, a child might only be able to flex (bend) the hips, internally rotate (turn in) the legs, and adduct them (bring the legs together). This will interfere with standing straight. Or a child might only be able to flex the elbow with the wrist and fingers flexed, too. This will interfere with self-feeding. We can try to improve these movements by helping the inactive muscles become more active. We might not be able to correct the problem totally because the original insult to the brain that caused the cerebral palsy might continue to limit the use of some muscles.

The examples that follow show how parents can help children with different functional limitations learn new skills at home, following some basic principles of NDT:

- Specific movement impairments that interfere with the skill the child is trying to perform must be evaluated and treated.

- Alignment of the segments of the body must be ideal for muscles to work their best and for the eyes to be used for learning.

- Key points of control (where parents put their hands) help the child move more efficiently and have more normal sensations of movement.

Examples

1. This 6-year-old boy has spastic quadriplegia. He can move only by rolling on the floor. Sitting in a chair is possible if he has support on the side of his trunk and head, a seat belt, and straps across his feet. He can stand if someone holds him up, but he always stands on his toes with his legs crossed. He can reach for toys and sometimes grasp and hold them if they are small enough. He often is frustrated because he wants to play with all kinds of toys. He can make only vowel sounds, and his few words are comprehensible only to his family. This little boy likes to be around other children and tries very hard to play and participate at school. His parents want him to be able to play with more kinds of toys and eventually to use a computer. It will be important that he learn to open his hands, reach forward, and bring his hands together. Some suggestions for parents:

Activity: Preparing the child's back and shoulders to be in a good position for reaching forward

Method: Seat the child on a small chair or bench and hold the child around the ribcage. If the child needs more support, use his adaptive chair. Sit in front of the child. Move your fingers that are on the back of his ribcage toward you to help him straighten up his back. Also, it usually helps to turn (rotate) his trunk to one side to help straighten him up. Then he can learn to move rather quickly from the midline position to the side and back again.

Next, press gently but firmly down over the tops of his shoulders so that he no longer hunches up his shoulders (looks like he is shrugging). It is easier for him to bring his arms forward if his shoulders aren't hunched up. Help guide his arms forward, usually by holding above his elbows (pulling at his hands usually makes the problem worse; he stiffens and pulls back away from you).

The next idea sounds odd, but it usually works. While still holding above the elbow or both elbows, rapidly wiggle the arm back and forth or up and down as if you were shaking apples off the limb of a tree. This very rapid movement usually makes most children much less stiff. Now you might be able to let go above the elbow and hold his wrist and a little bit into the bottom of the palm of his hand. It is critical in most instances to stay very near the wrist. If you get too far into the palm of his hand, he usually will close his hand tightly. While holding the wrist, give your child the desired toy. Press it firmly into his hand so that he can shape his hand around it. You will want to start with smaller toys and work up to larger ones.

2. This 9-year-old girl has diplegia. She can stand alone briefly and can walk with crutches but cannot walk independently. Because of some visual impairments, it's hard for her to look at objects with both eyes moving together. She has trouble correctly judging depth and distance. When she reads, she holds the book close to her face and looks at it out of the corners of her eyes. Her parents want her to be able to walk short distances independently, at least across a room so she can move more quickly and easily in a house, classroom, and eventually a workplace. She tends to walk with her hips and knees bent, hips turned in, and knees brushing against each other. Her heels don't ever seem to touch the ground, although she is not up on her toes. She takes very short steps and gets tired after walking through the hallways at school or in a store. Some suggestions for parents:

Activity: Standing straighter and taking a step

Method: Have the child stand in the middle of the room where she can't hold onto anything. (Remember, this is a child who can stand alone briefly. Children with diplegia will always rely on their arms rather than their legs when given a chance.) Sit or kneel behind the child on the floor. Hold around the front of her thighs just above her knees. You might want to put your shoulder against her buttocks to support her hips to stay straight. Ask her to push her feet down into the floor as long as she can. This should cause her to straighten her hips and knees actively. Don't say, "Straighten up"; say, "Push your feet into the floor as long as you can." The straighter she gets, the more she should be able to help you turn her feet out slightly and keep her knees apart. Now, lightly hold the flat palms of your hands on the sides of her hips. When you feel that she is standing securely, let go and see how long she can stand alone. After she can stand alone confidently for several seconds, ask for a step or two. You probably will want to put your hands back on the sides of her hips when she practices this.

3. This 6-year-old child has hemiplegia. He is able to walk, run, and climb stairs and curbs. He uses his left hand to help his more skillful right hand with such activities as holding down paper when he writes, throwing a large ball, getting undressed, and holding toys in place. He is having trouble at school carrying his lunch tray because his left arm flexes (bends) too much at the elbow and wrist. He cannot turn the palm of his hand up (this movement takes place in the forearm). Some suggestions for parents:

Activity: Carrying a large book across the room at home

Method: Carrying the book allows the child to practice carrying an object similar in weight and size to the cafeteria tray without the fear that dropping it will make a mess. If necessary, prepare the child's back and arm the same way as with the child who has spastic quadriplegia (example 1). Rest the child's left forearm on a tabletop as he is sitting or standing. Ask him to lean sideways behind the table, across the left arm. While he does this, roll his forearm so that the top of his hand and forearm come nearer the table while the palm of the hand begins to face the ceiling. Have him then hold the book with both arms while his forearms still rest against the table. After he can do this, have him try to pick the book up from the table. Start with a lighter-weight book and work up to a heavier one. Only when he can stand and hold the book comfortably should he try to walk with it. Don't wait until he can hold it perfectly; his left arm probably will never look like his right arm.

For more clarification of Neuro-Developmental Treatment (NDT) theory and how it influences therapy for children, see Article 1.2 by Judith Bierman, titled "Philosophy, Theory, and Principles: The What, Why, and How of NDT."

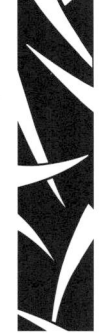

The Unique Physical Challenges of Children With Hypotonia

Marcia Stamer, PT

Hypotonia (low muscle tone) results from many different causes. Children with cerebral palsy usually (but not always) are hypotonic as babies and could develop athetosis (wide-range, uncontrolled movements), ataxia (balance and coordination problems), or even spasticity as they grow older. Hypotonia is common throughout life in children with a wide range of genetic disorders. Children with visual impairments often have low muscle tone, as do children with forms of muscular dystrophies and atrophies. These children don't look and move exactly the same way because their disorders are so different. Those who are very much affected have such a hard time moving that they don't move at all. Those who are mildly affected have trouble only with very hard skills such as playing a musical instrument, running, or kicking a soccer ball. Yet there are several common features of how children with hypotonia typically move. Some predictable characteristics are:

- Some difficulty making groups of muscles work together, especially when the muscles have to hold a contraction for periods of time. After I explained this to one father, he said, "It seems, then, that it would be easier for my son to be a boxer, not a wrestler." That's it! His son could make muscles contract long enough for the punch in boxing but not long enough for a wrestling hold.
- Delay in starting a movement. Once the movement is started, the child might be strong enough or able to use the correct muscles to perform the movement.
- Locking certain joints in positions of extension to substitute for insufficient muscle activity, or spreading the arms and legs wide apart to hold themselves up or to move between postures. These compensations make some movements possible but eventually interfere with the achievement of more skillful movements.

For example, a 12-month-old child can lie on her stomach, roll over and over, and scoot and wiggle around the floor but can't really crawl on her belly yet. When she is on her stomach, she often rests her head back on her spine and looks up toward the ceiling. She can sit if she is placed in a sitting position, will spread her legs apart, then lie down between them to get down on her stomach. She can stand only if someone holds her firmly around her trunk and holds her knees straight for her. She can pick up toys, but often they drop out of her hands as she tries to play with them. Her hands feel soft and mushy, as if they have no strength. She makes very few sounds, but you know which of her sounds indicate pleasure and displeasure. She clearly communicates yes and no with sounds and body language.

Neuro-Developmental Treatment (NDT) Principles

The following activities suggest ways you can use NDT principles and suggestions to help your child with hypotonia.

- **NDT Principle:** Specific movement impairments that interfere with the skill the child is trying to perform must be evaluated and treated. For example, weak trunk muscles that interfere with postural control can be strengthened with certain activities.

    Activity: Bouncing the child on your knees

    Method: Play a game with a nursery rhyme while you bounce your child on your knees. Have her sit on your knees facing you as you hold around her ribs firmly but not too tightly. Your hands help hold her back straight. Choose a medium pace for the rhythm of the nursery rhyme, matched with your bouncing. It is very important that you bounce her just enough to help her want to sit up straight. Don't let her head flop around. You can make sure this doesn't happen by looking her straight in the eyes as you talk so that she looks straight ahead at you. (You might need to lean back to get down to her level). If she can't hold her head up well enough for the bouncing activity, then sit her on your lap with her back and head against your chest as you read her a story, giving her a chance to hold her head up alone from time to time.

- **NDT Principle:** Alignment of the segments of the body must be ideal for muscles to work their best and for the eyes to be used for learning.

    Activity: Looking at toys, faces, or food that is motivating to your child

    Method: After the bouncing activity, sit your child in his high chair. It is critical that his back be straight and that he holds his head up so that he can look straight ahead and use his eyes for learning, especially if vision also is a problem. It is well worth your time and your therapist's time to explore many ways to support your child in the high chair so that he can use his eyes to look at you, at toys, and at food as much as possible. You can tilt the chair slightly backward, provide support around the belly with a wide, soft belt, or give support along the sides of the child's trunk and legs with foam inserts or rolled towels.

- **NDT Principle:** Learning movement skills is an active process that involves motivation and desire on the child's part as well as the ability to see, feel, and move.

   Activity: With your child sitting in a well-aligned position, present favorite toys, faces, or food in front of her.

   Method: Sing a song. Make the toys move. Help her touch your face, the food, or the toy. Give her praise and encouragement to keep looking at whatever you are showing her. Usually, the more a child uses her eyes to hold a gaze, the better her whole posture will be in sitting. Keep checking that her position in the high chair is ideal. Readjust as needed. Once she looks at you or a toy for a second or two, help her look at another face or toy by moving it slightly while the first stays still. While doing this, you should be directly in front of the high chair tray so that she doesn't have to look up or down. Touch her often and firmly to help her keep looking at you. After she is able to look from one toy or face to another, then you can start teaching her to choose between the two.

For more clarification of Neuro-Developmental Treatment (NDT) theory and how it influences therapy for children, see Article 1.2 by Judith Bierman, titled "Philosophy, Theory, and Principles: The What, Why, and How of NDT."

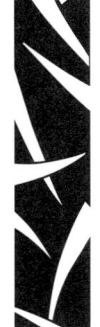

The Unique Physical Challenges of Children With Athetosis

Marcia Stamer, PT

Children with the athetoid type of cerebral palsy show distinct problems in their postures and movements. Athetosis (from Greek, meaning *not stationary*) is characterized by wide-range, uncontrolled movements that often get worse the harder the child tries to do something. Athetosis might be the only type of cerebral palsy your child has, or it might be present in combination with spastic cerebral palsy. Occasionally, athetosis occurs with ataxia.

Athetoid movements can be mild, but more commonly the movement disorder is severe. Children with athetosis often cannot sit, walk, talk, or hold onto objects, yet these children usually have average or above-average intelligence, with or without learning disabilities. Because they have so many movement problems and so many different ways of moving, parents and therapists often are at a loss when trying to help children with athetosis learn functional movement skills. In fact, one of the most difficult problems is that they often perform the same skill with a different movement from one time to the next. So how do we help them?

In observing children with athetosis, I find that there are certain consistencies in their movements and strategies that sometimes help them learn a skill but oftentimes don't. Some of the common ways that children with athetosis move include:

- Moving the head and eyes to one side as a way to start movement anywhere in the body. This occurs most frequently when the child is attempting to reach for something. The child turns her head away from the arm that is reaching. This does help the arm reach, but the price the child pays is that she can't see what she's reaching for.

- Using only movements that either totally extend (straighten) or flex (bend) parts of the body. The child can't seem to bend one joint while straightening another (i.e., when grasping a spoon, the wrist should extend while the fingers flex). In addition, when the child uses extension, which usually is the way children with athetosis move, it is usually with very large, fast movements while the head is turned to one side. If the child pushes and extends hard enough with the head turned to the side, the back starts to bend to one side only.

- Large-range movements of jaw opening and closing, which the child cannot control when he eats or tries to make sounds. He either opens the jaw forcefully, usually with the tongue sticking out, or clamps his mouth shut. He usually needs to drop his head down to clamp the jaw shut.

- Breathing is not coordinated with attempts to make sounds or talk. The child might be very bright but unable to make sounds or talk.

Because of the severe problems that most children with athetosis have, many are unable to do some very necessary skills, such as feeding themselves. If we look more closely at this skill, we can understand why it causes such great difficulties. Let's say that the child is sitting in her wheelchair or another chair that supports her sitting posture well. There is a plate in front of her with green beans. You stab two small green beans and place the fork in her hand. She is able to hold onto the fork, at least for awhile. What happens next is one of two things: She either turns her head and eyes to one side and completely opens her jaw as the hand with the fork waves around in front of her, or she drops her head forward and can't bend her elbow to bring the fork to her mouth. Either way she does it, she is unable to feed herself. In addition, the harder she tries, the worse it gets (this is almost always true of children with athetosis).

Neuro-Developmental Treatment (NDT) Principles

The following activities suggest ways parents can use NDT principles and suggestions to help their child with athetosis:

- **NDT Principle:** Specific movement impairments that interfere with the skill the child is trying to perform must be evaluated and treated.

  Activity: Playing a game that teaches the child how to bend the elbow joint while holding his head straight in the middle. (I have found that almost all children with athetosis can learn at least to hold the head closer to the middle so that they can see what they are reaching for. This takes a lot of practice.)

  Method: Play a game with your child such as a beanbag toss. Keep score. It's more fun to play with Dad, Mom, a sibling, or a friend. Help the child hold his head up and in the middle while he sits, with your help, on a chair where you can sit behind him. Your therapist might have ideas for the best way to do this, or you might be able to show the therapist where it's best to hold the child. Your child's job is to look at the beanbag while someone places it in his hand (he doesn't have to reach for it yet). To score points in the game, he only has to look at what is in his hand as you help hold his head in place. Even if he can't keep his head right in the middle, give him points if he still can look at what is in his hand as he holds it. Of course, you will want to help him throw it at a target for fun.

- **NDT Principles:** Stability of the head, eyes, and trunk allow for more skilled movements of the arms and legs. Therapy includes hands-on facilitation of movement that must be decreased as the child takes over the movement. The goal of therapy always is a functional skill.

   Activity: Continue the above game, making it more challenging.

- **Method:** Try to decrease your support to the child's head. You might be able to hold somewhere around her trunk—at the shoulders or around the waist. She still must look at the beanbag while you place it in her hand, or perhaps now she can assist with the reach and/or grasp. After she can do this, ask her to hold the beanbag and touch her nose with it before throwing it. Here, she scores points for holding her head and eyes up straight and close enough to the middle that she can see the beanbag at all times (except when it's very close to her nose!). Your goal is for her to improve her ability to hold her head up and close to the middle while she bends her elbow and brings her hand to her nose (close to her mouth). Next, see if she can do the same thing when sitting in her wheelchair or other supportive chair. Finally, when she practices enough that this movement becomes easier, try putting food on a fork and ask her to bring it to her mouth.

Note: Many children with athetosis learn well with games that are similar to the skill you want to teach them but don't involve the emotional effort of trying the skill itself. It seems that they can generalize movement patterns well from one situation to another. And because they don't do well when they are trying so hard to reach a real goal (like putting food into the mouth), it's easier to practice the movement with a game that is fun and not so emotionally charged.

For more clarification of Neuro-Developmental Treatment (NDT) theory and how it influences therapy for children, see Article 1.2 by Judith Bierman, titled "Philosophy, Theory, and Principles: The What, Why, and How of NDT."

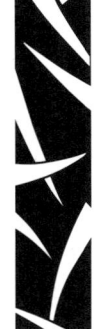

The Unique Physical Challenges of Children With Ataxia

Marcia Stamer, PT

Children with ataxic cerebral palsy have several very distinct characteristics compared with other children with cerebral palsy. First, ataxia often is not diagnosed as early as other types of cerebral palsy because children who have ataxia do not show movement problems that are obvious to parents until they are older. They are unlike children with spastic cerebral palsy who are stiff and delayed in sitting, reaching for toys, and making sounds. They differ from children with athetoid cerebral palsy who show uncontrolled, large-range movements and are very delayed in most motor skills.

Instead, babies who will become ataxic sometimes appear to be strong and might develop some of their motor skills on time. But typically, their parents notice some distinct problems that are difficult to understand and often take longer to figure out than the movement problems of children with other types of cerebral palsy. To complicate matters, many children with cerebral palsy have mixtures of spastic diplegia and ataxia, or athetosis and ataxia. I also have seen children who are spastic, athetoid, and ataxic! Characteristics of ataxia can include a combination of behaviors:

- Looking at people or toys for only short periods of time
- Reaching and holding toys, but only by grabbing them hard, stuffing them in their mouths, biting, and throwing them. Although all babies do these things to a certain extent, children with ataxia retain these behaviors while others their age move on to more exploring and manipulating.
- Making very few sounds
- Stuffing excessive amounts of food into the mouth or storing it there instead of swallowing
- Reacting too much and too long to loud sounds or sudden changes in lighting
- Motor delays, appearing later rather than sooner, especially movements such as getting in and out of sitting or standing
- Sometimes too floppy or too stiff (only when scared), and other times all right
- Tremoring in some part of the body, but not all the time
- Reacting slowly or clumsily when losing balance
- Not watching where he is going, staring into space when moving, and not noticing anything in the room

One of the reasons for these difficulties is that children with ataxia have trouble processing and using information from one or more of the sensory systems. Sensory systems include vision, taste, smell, hearing, and touch. Children can interpret these sensations (as well as some others) as meaningful only when the brain is maturing normally. For example, information from joints and muscles tells us the position of our arms, head, legs, and body and must be integrated with visual input. Children with ataxia can see, but they don't always understand what they see. The trouble isn't with the eyes but how the brain uses what the eyes see. Also, they don't always feel where their bodies are as they move. In addition to their sensory problems, they often have trouble with motor control, such as being able to move quickly or at the right time. Balance reactions happen too slowly or not at all.

Children with ataxia don't watch where they are going and don't look down, so they fall a lot. They especially have trouble looking down when they move. They reach too far for a toy (overshoot) or not far enough (undershoot). They walk with feet spread wide apart to help with balance. Because they often are very afraid of movement, they might refuse to try a movement, or they might do just the opposite, moving as fast as they can but with no control.

For example, a child walks by herself and can climb stairs when she holds onto a rail or someone's hand. She can step up the curb on the sidewalk near her house without holding onto anything. But she can't walk up the two steps into her house unless her parents help her, because there is no handrail on these steps. This is confusing to her parents because the steps aren't as high as the curb, which she can do without holding on. However, the height of the step isn't the problem, because her legs are strong. The problem is that the steps are narrow (both the width and depth), whereas the curb steps up to a wide sidewalk. She probably is unable to express her fear that she can't manage the narrow spaces on the stair steps without losing her balance. Somehow she knows that she has poor balance and depth perception. This is very typical of children with ataxia. They seem to be able to do some things (such as the high curb) and not others (such as the lower steps) that we think they should be able to do.

All of these problems can be traced to the area of the brain known as the cerebellum. This area seems to be responsible for well-timed movement, for the memory of movement, and for the processing of many different sensations. Often, even modern brain scans and imaging don't show where the problem is, so the doctor has to make a diagnosis based on observable signs as described previously. But parents and their team of professionals can make sense of the difficulties that children are having by thinking about their specific problems and figuring out why.

Neuro-Developmental Treatment (NDT) Principles

The following activities suggest ways parents can use NDT principles to help their child with ataxia.

- **NDT Principle:** Specific movement impairments that interfere with the skill the child is trying to perform must be evaluated and treated. Learning a movement skill first requires the use of information from the sensory systems.

  Activity: Feeling the body position in space while standing and enhancing the visual information for standing and stepping up

  Method: Have the child stand in front of a stair step. Place brightly colored tape on the edge of each step. Ask your child to look at the tape while you place your hands firmly on top of his shoulders. When he is standing straight, you also can push firmly down on his shoulders toward the ground. Ask him to step up while you hold him firmly while pushing down through his shoulders.

- **NDT Principle:** Because the outcome of therapy is function, activity in therapy always should end with practice of the functional skill desired.

  Activity: Walking up steps with assistance

  Method: You might need to hold your child firmly to step up the steps until she is not so afraid. But if you hold her hands, she probably won't want to let go. Instead, hold her firmly around her waist or over the top of her shoulders as she steps up. If she leans back toward you, go around the front and help her from there. In climbing steps, she should lean forward to go up, not backward.

- **NDT Principle:** Therapy includes hands-on facilitation of movement but also includes the gradual withdrawal of assistance as the child takes over the movement.

  Activity: Climbing the steps into the house independently

  Method: This is a critical step in helping a child with ataxia learn a skill. Practice holding him as in the example above, but lighten your touch as he learns the movement, or touch him firmly as he begins, then let go after he starts the movement. Be ready to catch him if he loses his balance.

Note: In practicing skills with children who are ataxic, I find it necessary to practice the real thing. Practicing on something else is nothing like the steps at home. This is clearly different from children with other types of cerebral palsy who might be able to generalize new skills to similar but not identical situations. I don't know exactly why this is true, but I suspect that it is because children with ataxia have several problems with motor learning (the cerebellum seems to be a primary center for motor learning).

For more clarification of Neuro-Developmental Treatment (NDT) theory and how it influences therapy for children, see Article 1.2 by Judith Bierman, titled "Philosophy, Theory, and Principles: The What, Why, and How of NDT."

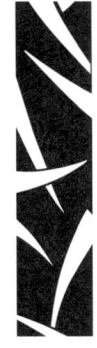

Making Movement Easier Through Touch
Regi Boehme, OTR

Have you every wondered what therapists' hands are doing as we touch your child during therapy? It's no secret. Our hands are "talking" to your child about how to make movement easier. Our hands speak a language called *levels of touch*. If we actually could hear the language of touch, it would sound like conversations from many different countries because there are so many different ways to touch and messages that our touch can give.

For example, sometimes your child is trying very hard to move but his body feels heavy. Movement can feel like a struggle. The body is confused about which muscles to use. In this case, our touch helps by supporting some of the body weight. We also speak to the body, telling it to push against the floor. Each time your child pushes against the supporting surface, his body gets taller and lighter. Movement gets easier. Then, your child can begin to feel which muscles to use. He will feel less frustrated and eventually movement will feel pleasurable. Our goal always is to help your child learn to move independently without the language of our touch.

Sometimes your child is trying very hard to move but feels stuck in one spot. It feels as if she is glued to the floor. Then our touch gently helps your child shift her weight safely from one limb to another. This allows the unweighted limb the freedom to change positions or move forward. It's just like when you are walking. You have to transfer your body weight to one leg so you can move the other leg forward. As we help your child learn weight shifting, the child no longer will feel glued to the floor.

Sometimes your child is trying to move but the muscles get stiff. When the muscles around the joints get stiff, the joints can't bend or straighten. Your child might feel trapped in his body when the joints can't move. Our touch can tell your child's body to relax. We can rock the stiff areas gently until the muscles relax. We can keep the muscles soft and relaxed by continuing small rocking motions as your child is moving. These small rocking motions are like miniature weight shifts.

Sometimes your child wants to move but can't because she's unable to make the muscles active. Muscle activity is important for movement so is muscle strength and muscle endurance. We can't move easily and safely without activity, strength, and endurance. Some children have weak muscles, and other children have muscles that respond very slowly to stimulation. In either case, our touch can help wake up the muscles with massage, pressure, or light tapping directly on the muscles. We might use toys that are brightly colored and make sounds to stimulate your child and increase his desire to attempt to move. The more attempts he makes, the stronger he will get.

Although some children get stiff, your child might be highly flexible. Highly flexible children feel very heavy when you lift them. This is because they can't support their own body weight. Some children even have difficulty lifting their head. Highly flexible children usually have weak muscles. They respond well to careful bouncing on a ball or in our lap. Sometimes, we rub them with a terrycloth towel to wake up their muscles.

In therapy, we sometimes passively start a movement through our touch, then wait a long time for your child to finish the movement. Waiting is important. Often, there is a delay between your child's desire to move and her ability to move.

Or, we might encourage your child to start moving while we maintain contact with his body and move with him. We do this for two reasons. We want to keep your child safe from injuries, and we want to be ready if he needs a little help.

We can use the language of touch to lengthen muscles that have become short over time. When we use touch to lengthen a muscle, we don't stretch it forcibly, because stretching can be uncomfortable. We straighten the muscle until we feel the first hint of resistance. We wait there until the muscle gets softer. Then, through our touch, we check to feel whether the muscle is more flexible. If it is, we move the limb a little farther until we feel a little resistance. We keep repeating this process as long as your child is comfortable. Sometimes during the waiting period we add a little rocking motion to help the muscle relax.

These are some examples of the language of touch. We can vary our pressure from light to medium to firm-touch contact. How much pressure we give depends on how much support your child needs and how well she feels information in her muscles and joints. We can vary the speed of the movement as we touch. We use the speed that is most like the natural rhythm of your child's movement. We move with your child so that your child feels that moving is safe.

The language of touch is respectful, loving, and safe, yet some children have difficulty being touched. There are many reasons for this difficulty. Some children need to feel that they are in control of their body. We try very hard to avoid imposing movement on children. They learn best by directing their own movements. When their preferred way of moving is creating barriers to further progress, then our touch will guide them in the direction of more mature movement patterns.

Some children do not tolerate touch to their skin. We adapt by touching them while they are fully clothed. What we cannot see, we can feel. Some children have a general intolerance for touch and movement. It seems to confuse them. We then might use indirect touch such as swinging in a hammock, brushing their body through their clothes, or letting them play with a hand-held vibrator. This helps the sensory systems organize so that your child can experience touch with more ease.

The language of our touch is our tool for helping your child experience his body positively and to explore his world successfully. Our goal for each child is to reach his or her full potential. Gentle touch is the language of acceptance, encouragement, and trust.

Therapists who use the Neuro-Developmental Treatment (NDT) approach are concerned about teaching functional skills. But we first observe what movements the child can do. We then analyze the areas of movement difficulties by observing with our eyes and feeling with our hands. By guiding the correct movements, therapists find that the child can move in more functional ways. We remove our guidance as the child performs the skill more independently, efficiently, and confidently.

Parents, naturally, have the most familiar and loving touch for their children. Moving your child slowly helps her feel her body motions through your body motions. The same thing happens when you are helping your child move. When you move slowly, she can feel movement more clearly. Slow movement gives her time to respond, for example, by putting her arm out to meet the floor or by moving her head back in line with her trunk. My husband John always says, "The slower you go, the faster you get there." He's referring to the child's ability to develop independent movement skills over time.

It's important to wait for a response when you are moving, playing, or helping your child with self-care. It's hard to know how much help a child really needs. Children often can do more than we realize. It just takes them more time. In addition, they might need time to learn the various pieces of a skill and to practice one piece at a time. For example, your child might be able to grasp a spoon, and need help only with filling the spoon and bringing it to his mouth. When you assist him slowly, you might notice that he needs only a little help with the weight of his arm. You can cradle your child's arm as if you are a sling supporting the weight while he moves it by himself. In this situation, the less you do, the more he does. Each movement he does on his own is a stepping stone toward independence.

It is not always possible to move slowly and consciously with a child. Our days are filled with many demands and little leisure time. Having a child with special needs increases the demands of everyday life. But these small messages you give through your touch can add up eventually to better balance and control.

The best time to work with your child is when you feel relaxed. Early evenings or weekends might be your most relaxed time. The rest of the time, your child needs to feel the love of a parental touch. The touch of unconditional love, without expectation, is a wonderful way to touch your child.

Rubbing or stroking the body can improve a child's awareness of those body parts that she is not yet ready to use independently. This unconditional touch gives the message, "I love your body. I love the way it feels." At the same time, it offers the child a sense of her whole body and prepares her for tolerating and understanding future movements.

For example, some children have difficulty getting onto their feet or using their feet to change positions. Massage will maintain good circulation and reduce hypersensitivity to standing or other forms of movement. The same is true for the rest of the body. Some children are unable to take weight through their arms or hands. Massaging and gently straightening each finger and thumb can help these children enjoy the feeling of movement and touch in their hands. You can incorporate stroking and rubbing into bath time or washing the face and hands after meals.

We therapists sometimes ask you to carry over an exercise program at home. If your child is receiving more than one therapy, you might have to do many things at home with your child. It's important to describe your daily activities to us and tell us what other therapists have asked you to do. Ask us which exercise is the most important. Ask us to demonstrate it on you, so that you feel the quality of touch. Practice on your therapists.

Protect your own energy and normal family time. Integrate home-centered therapy into the natural rhythm and timing of the rest of the family. In addition, each child has his or her own rhythm and timing for meals, sleep, and play. Always respect and protect this internal rhythm.

Please refer to Article 5.6, "Caring Strokes for Little Folks: Therapeutic Pediatric Massage."

For more clarification of Neuro-Developmental Treatment (NDT) theory and how it influences therapy for children, see Article 1.2 by Judith Bierman, titled "Philosophy, Theory, and Principles: The What, Why, and How of NDT."

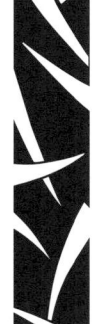

Touching Is Fun! Helping Children Learn to Use Their Hands

Lezlie Adler, M.A., OTR, FMOT

Parents want children to learn to take care of themselves. The ability to do that depends a lot on how well they use their hands to manipulate objects in their environment. Manipulation is a learned skill that develops as children gain motor control over the smaller parts of their body, begin to understand sensations from their own body and the world around them, and develop the desire to explore their environment actively. Parents of children with movement problems, sensory processing disorders, or mental impairment often ask how they can help their children improve their hand skills. There is no simple answer. The components of purposeful hand function are (a) motor control, (b) sensory processing, and (c) motivation—the desire to do and learn. Even when children's motor skills or understanding are limited, learning to use their hands is really important, a key to independence in daily living activities, school, and play.

Children learn a lot about how their hands work from experiences that don't include manipulation. The very first step is to recognize that they have hands! This is accomplished when they see their hands at the ends of their arms or feel them.

The asymmetrical tonic neck reflex pattern can give a child his first visual exposure to his hands. When a child turns his head, the arm on the face side straightens so that the hand is in clear sight. Fortunately, even the very young child can see clearly to the end of his hand. Turning the head to both sides lets the child know he has two hands!

When a young child sucks on her thumb or fingers or puts a different part in her mouth (even her whole hand!), she gains a little bit more information about her hand, fingers, and palm by feeling those sensations of sucking or biting.

When a child moves his hands over different parts of his body, he receives double the information. If he is holding a toy, he not only learns about the toy but also how to use his hands.

Another way a child learns to use her arms and hands without putting anything in them is when she lifts her head up and places weight first on her forearms and then on her hands as she pushes up higher with straight elbows and flat hands on the surface. At first, she holds her arms and hands close to her body but with increasing control, she can move them farther away. As she gains more control of her head and trunk, she will begin to move her arms through space or use her arms and hands purposefully to push her body up off the floor. This pushing with the hands puts lots of pressure on them, making the child very aware of how she can use her hands to support her body.

The more opportunities children have to move on the floor, the more information they get about their hands. Rolling to the side or all the way over helps children learn to place their arms in different positions and hold them there. Pushing up and down from elbows to straight arms, commando crawling, moving from the back or stomach to sit, rocking on hands and knees, bear walking, and finally, coming up to stand all are ways children learn to use arms and hands for transitional movements (moving from one position to another).

Transitional movements are wonderful developmental opportunities for children to get lots of sensory information from muscles, bones, and skin. This essential information tells children how and where they can position their arms and hands, how they can use arms and hands together or separately, and how to use one arm for control and the other for manipulation. Children's abilities to gain control over their bodies and learn to move through space are essential elements for learning to use their hands.

Just as important as motor control is the understanding of sensation, which helps the child learn how to hold, transport (move), and release objects. The first sensations that are most helpful to the infant are vision, touch, and pressure. In fact, children use their eyes first to grasp the environment, learning much information about how to hold and manipulate objects before touching them. When a child begins to hold and touch things, that additional information from touch and pressure helps develop the important process of accommodation.

Accommodation is the way the hands mold around differently shaped objects. To accommodate appropriately, the child's hands must open and close easily, and muscles of the wrist and hand must work in different combinations to move the bones and joints into a wide variety of positions. How the object feels (size, weight, shape, etc.) is what drives these movements. The brain interprets these sensations so as to select the correct grasp. The best way for children to learn to hold and manipulate objects is by practice. They want to touch everything! They grab, drop, squeeze, turn, and bang things. Each action gives them a little more information about how their hands work and what they can do. This is the major way children learn to receive sensory input, process it, and practice using their hands in different ways.

Finally, this motivation, this drive for motor control and desire for sensory information, comes from within the child. It is created by cognition and curiosity and is essential for learning to use the hands purposefully. Use of the arms and hands for support and transitional movements represents well-established patterns in the nervous system. Curiosity that comes from the child is the overlay on those patterns. The transition of the use of arms and hands from weight-bearing to purposeful action is a major jump needed for the development of a wide variety of hand movements. These include prehension patterns (grasping an object so that it can be used for its intended purpose) and in-hand manipulation (moving an object within the palm and/or fingers of one hand, such as turning a pencil over in one hand to use the eraser).

Neuro-Developmental Treatment (NDT) Principles

NDT principles provide guidelines for simple ideas to help children learn to use their hands purposefully. Most of these suggestions apply to young children, but you easily can adapt many of them for older children and adolescents. You can incorporate them into everyday play activities.

- **NDT Principle:** The development of motor control begins with the central part of the body (head, trunk, and pelvis) as a foundation for controlling more distal parts (arms and hands, legs and feet).

  Activity: Handling and positioning

  Method: When you are playing with your child or trying to encourage hand use, first get alignment of the head, trunk, and pelvis before you present something to touch. You can achieve this in a seating system or on your lap using your own body to give alignment and support, if necessary. This support will help the child's arms move away from the trunk. Hold the toy far enough away to encourage your child to reach for it.

- **NDT Principle:** The ability to learn new motor behaviors depends on the opportunity for sensation, movement, and practice.

  Activity: Sensory exploration of touch and pressure

  Method: You can provide sensory information about molding and shaping by doing something as simple as holding and squeezing your child's hand. First wrap your hand around your child's hand and give gentle pressure or squeeze and hold. Move your fingers into the palm, then scoop or shape the palm and gently tug on each of the fingers. This is a good way to prepare the hands of children who can't give themselves this type of sensory input, especially just before you place an object in the hand or offer a toy to be reached for and touched.

- **Principle:** Motor control of the arms and hands begins with their use in weight bearing and transitional movements prior to intentional use in space.

  Activity: Weight bearing and weight shifting through the hands

  Method: Place a towel roll under your child's armpits or a pillow or wedge under the trunk when the child is lying in prone, propping on forearms, or pushing up on extended arms with open hands. Or simply place your hand flat against your child's hand, in any position, and push gently up through the hand into the wrist, making sure the hand stays in the middle. You also can place your child's open hands together, or put one of the child's hands on her thigh or forearm, pushing down so that the child can feel the pressure on her open hand. This provides the feeling of a big, open hand that is important for release as well as grasp.

- **NDT Principle:** Sensory information is essential to developing new motor behaviors.

  Activity: Using vision as the first "hand" to prehend (grasp)

  Method: Make sure your child looks at an object before reaching and playing with it, in order to lay the foundation for eye-hand coordination. If head control is a problem (falling forward, backward, or to the side), help by supporting the head at its base, lifting it up, and directing the child's face toward the activity. You can do this by making a *U* with your index finger and thumb, then lining them up with the bottom of your child's ears.

- **NDT Principle:** Development of skill acquisition depends on many systems providing information with opportunities to interact with the environment.

  Activity: Choice of multisensory toys and objects

  Method: Select objects and toys that provide lots of sensory input for your child to experience. Toys can feel soft, hard, rough, smooth, wet, dry, cold, or warm, and make noise easily. Toys that let the child receive lots of different types of sensory input are more valuable than those that must be manipulated in a special way for a single purpose. Variety is the most important element. The more experiences the child has, the more opportunities there are for learning, and the more willing the child will be to explore.

- **NDT Principle:** Motor learning is best achieved by engaging in activities that have purpose and meaning to the person.

Activity: Learning accommodation through play

Method: Think about objects and activities that would be novel and interesting to your child and spark natural curiosity. Children love playing with objects that Mom uses for cooking or that Dad uses to fix things. They will use these objects in different ways in imaginative play. For example, turkey basters, measuring cups, and funnels can be enjoyable bathtub toys. Children can use paintbrushes as spoons for snacks or to apply perfume or makeup. This variety is important because accommodation skills develop through opportunities to contour the hand around different-shaped objects.

Precautions

Don't force your child to use his or her hands. If the child appears to be frightened by a particular activity or object, stop and think about what might be causing that reaction. Try to adapt the activity so that it is more appealing, or allow alternatives for holding, such as the mouth, the foot, or the arm. Provide opportunities that are interesting and feel good. Remember that lots of different sensory inputs—especially vision, touch, and pressure—are the most interesting and important to most children.

Summary

Learning to use the hands purposefully depends on three primary components of development:

- motor control of the central part of the body (head and trunk), so that the arms and hands can be free from weight bearing and can move through space.
- understanding the sensations of vision, touch, and pressure that will lead to the process of accommodation.
- cognitive motivation and desire that will drive the child's natural curiosity to explore with the hands.

Parents and therapists can provide many structured activities for children to learn to use their hands. But self-initiated, intentional use of the hands depends on children's inner desire and willingness to explore. In other words, touching can be fun!

For more clarification of Neuro-Developmental Treatment (NDT) theory and how it influences therapy for children, see Article 1.2 by Judith Bierman, titled "Philosophy, Theory, and Principles: The What, Why, and How of NDT."

Handling With Care or Handling Carefully: Sensory Problems in Infants With Cerebral Palsy

Mary Hallway, OTR

Infants with cerebral palsy demonstrate movement disorders that interfere with their ability to participate in daily activities. Physical therapists, occupational therapists, and/or speech-language pathologists usually provide parents with special instructions, based on Neuro-Developmental Treatment (NDT), about how to position and handle their infants during lifting, carrying, bathing, dressing, and play. Therapists individualize these instructions to promote alignment and address the movement needs of each child.

Sometimes, in addition to their movement difficulties, these children have sensory processing problems in one or more of the sensory systems. This can influence how they respond to the environment and interact with caregivers (especially their handling during daily living activities). Current research has identified how important the sensory systems are for infants' motor development. These senses include visual (sight), tactile (touch), vestibular (movement), and proprioceptive (sensation from joints and muscles). This article describes signs of sensory problems in infants and suggests ways you can adjust your handling and positioning during daily activities to address both the sensory and motor needs of your child.

Current research indicates that infants can demonstrate sensory processing deficits in one or more of the sensory systems. Some underreact to sensory stimuli; others overreact. Some infants show both under- and overreactivity to certain sensory stimuli! The research identified behaviors in babies diagnosed with sensory problems, but these same behaviors (underreaction or overreaction to sensory input) also have been observed in babies with cerebral palsy.

Underreaction to Sensory Input

An infant with cerebral palsy who generally is underreactive to sensory input may appear to be a quiet, good baby and be difficult to excite and engage socially.

Babies who are underreactive to touch might respond slowly or not at all when touched, even to pain. Although they might have the oral-motor skills to begin eating solid foods, they have difficulties biting and chewing. They might not be aware of food left in their mouths. Older infants might crave and seek touch input by constantly putting objects in their mouths.

We can recognize tactile problems in infants with hemiplegia (where movement is affected on one side of the body more than the other) if the children ignore the affected arm and leg during play. These infants might not use both hands to explore their bodies (bringing hands together, hands to feet, and hands to mouth). They might not respond to being touched on the more affected side. Several studies have recorded problems localizing touch on both arms and feeling the difference between various objects in older children with hemiplegia.

Other studies found underresponsiveness to movement and proprioception (pressure sensations felt in the joints and muscles) in children with different types of cerebral palsy: increased muscle tone, athetosis (fluctuating tone), or ataxia (difficulties with steadiness and coordination). In early infancy, these children have difficulty adjusting their head, body, and arms when they are lifted and carried. These delayed adjustments also might be related to their motor difficulties. And yet these babies sometimes have a strong preference for movement activities such as bouncing, swinging, rocking, and roughhousing.

Overreaction to Sensory Input

An infant who generally is overreactive to sensory stimuli might pull away, cry, or be fearful in response to one or more types of sensory input.

Infants with cerebral palsy who overreact to touch might not like having their diapers or clothing changed, ears cleaned, hair washed or brushed, and/or being bathed and towel dried. These infants don't like to cuddle, might pull or arch away when held, and might cry during therapy sessions. They sometimes dislike being on different textured surfaces, such as carpet, sand, or grass. Their problems with changes in feeding are not related just to oral-motor control but to certain tactile elements. For example, changes in the bottle nipple, introduction to spoon feeding, or foods with new and unfamiliar textures can be very upsetting. Although they have the hand skills to feed themselves, babies with sensitive hands sometimes don't want to use their fingers. They dislike getting their hands messy during eating.

Babies who are overreactive to proprioception sometimes avoid taking weight on their arms and legs for crawling, pulling to stand, and walking. Their sensitivity seems to limit how much they move, although they have the motor skills to do so.

Some infants with increased muscle tone are unable to move around independently; therefore, they don't get much movement sensation (vestibular). They will feel insecure when new movements are introduced because of their difficulties with moving and controlling their bodies against gravity. Other infants react negatively to movement because of sensory problems, in addition to their movement difficulties. They become upset when they are handled in therapy or tipped backward to be put down in a crib or in the tub to have their hair washed. Riding in a car is unpleasant, as is swinging or roughhousing.

Some babies with cerebral palsy also demonstrate overreaction to sight and sound. They become distressed at household noises such as the vacuum cleaner, coffee grinder, leaf blower, or car engine. A baby who is overreactive to sights might turn away from looking at things that have a lot of detail, such as faces or a wall full of pictures. They might squint in response to light. Infants who are overreactive to both sight and sound sometimes become fussy when they go to the grocery store, mall, or restaurants—places that have too much or too many kinds of stimuli.

An infant with cerebral palsy who has difficulties in both sensory and movement development will benefit from a handling approach combining principles from both Neuro-Developmental Treatment (NDT) and Sensory Integration (SI) treatment. Parents can integrate both treatment approaches into handling during daily activities. Both emphasize how important it is for parents and other caregivers to be aware of the infant's responses, which indicate how the infant is receiving and processing the input. The primary goal is to give input that encourages and helps the baby interact and adapt. Parents and caregivers need to be aware of and eliminate or change input that causes a negative reaction.

The following activities combine both NDT and SI principles for handling infants who have both motor and sensory difficulties during daily activities. You and your child's therapist can decide which activities might benefit your child most.

Tips for Creating an Interactive Environment

Therapists and researchers have identified the following sensory inputs as either calming or exciting.

- **Touch:** Infants who are overreactive to touch during daily activities might be able to tolerate deep-pressure touch. Use light touch to stimulate infants who are underreactive. Both types of infants need a variety of touch experiences during play and other daily activities. Infants who react negatively to touch that is imposed might respond positively if allowed to initiate their own exploration of the textures.

- **Movement:** Many opportunities arise during daily activities for babies with cerebral palsy to receive a variety of movement sensations. Slow rhythmical movements (up and down or side to side) are relaxing to infants who react negatively to movement. Quick movements through a wide range (up and down, side to side, or in circles) are stimulating for those babies who are underreactive.

- **Visual Input:** Lighting in a room can be a source of overstimulation. Natural or low lighting might be tolerated better by infants who react negatively to light. You might need to alter the amount of visual stimuli in the environment by increasing or decreasing the amount of input.

- **Sound:** Infants who are overreactive to sound tolerate lower volume and rhythmic sound. Singing and other sounds with moderate volume will stimulate infants who need greater input.

Bathing

Bath time is a great time to introduce a variety of textures to infants who are underresponsive to touch. Wash your baby with sponges, wash cloths, and soft loofas and brushes. Try drying afterward with various textured towels, rubbing back and forth vigorously. Your baby who overreacts to touch might respond to being washed firmly with a terry towel or your hand, then wrapped or swaddled in a towel and dried with deep pressure on body parts (hugging while wrapped in the towel). Both underreactive and overreactive infants can benefit from an infant massage during their bathing routine (refer to Article 5.6, "Caring Strokes for Little Folks: Therapeutic Pediatric Massage").

Dressing

Incorporate specific movement sensations into dressing and undressing routines for infants who are underresponsive to movement. For example, you can transition your baby from sitting sideward to lying on the stomach while on your lap. This also will facilitate active head and trunk control throughout the dressing process. Support the child sitting sideward on your lap, then move the child down to prone (on the stomach) by bringing the child close to your body, placing your arm around the baby's backside, up under the arms, and across the chest. Place your other hand on the hip closest to you. Roll the baby to the stomach by turning the upper body first, allowing the hips and legs to follow (Figures 1a and 1b). Pull a shirt over the head by pulling it on from the back of the head to the front (a good idea for all infants). Insert the child's arms into the shirt, and pull it down by weight-shifting the child

Handling With Care or Handling Carefully: Sensory Problems in Infants With Cerebral Palsy

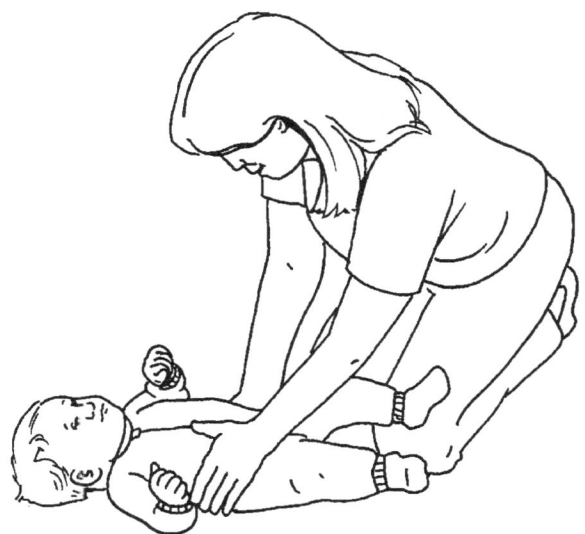

Figure 1a. Place one arm behind the baby, coming up under the arms and across the chest. Hold onto the upper arm. Place the other hand between the legs. Begin to rotate the baby to turn the child onto the stomach, leading with the arm and upper body first.

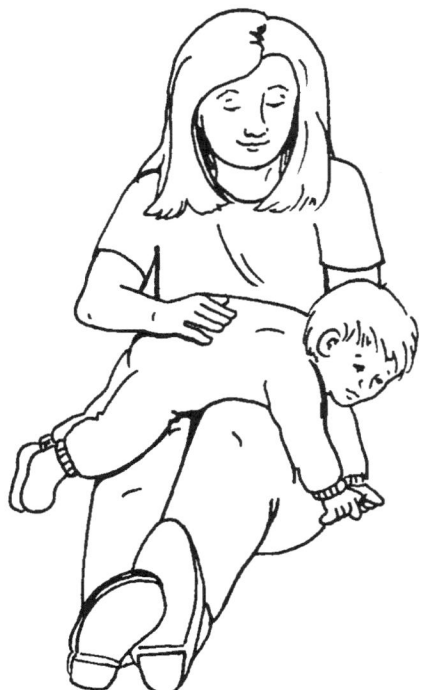

Figure 1b. Allow the baby's hips and legs to follow as you move the child into lying on the stomach. Weight shift the baby's body side to side with one hand on the back to facilitate adjustments with the baby's head and trunk sideways while pulling down the shirt.

from side to side. You also can put on pants using the weight-shifting technique.

Bring your baby back to sitting by placing your hand under the armpit closest to you and your other arm between the legs, with your hand on the stomach. Use that hand supporting the stomach to roll the child to the side and to shift the child's weight down toward his hips. At the same time, use your other hand to lift the child up to sitting while supporting his shoulders and head, if needed. The speed of the movement can vary depending on your baby's ability to adjust his head and body and respond to the movement (Figures 2a and 2b).

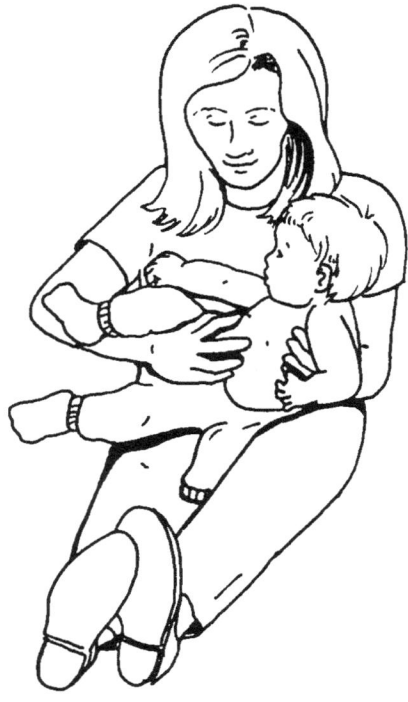

Figure 2a. Place one hand under the baby's armpit and one arm between the baby's legs with your hand on the stomach. Use the hand that supports the stomach to shift the baby's weight down toward the hips. At the same time, use your other hand to rotate the child up to sitting.

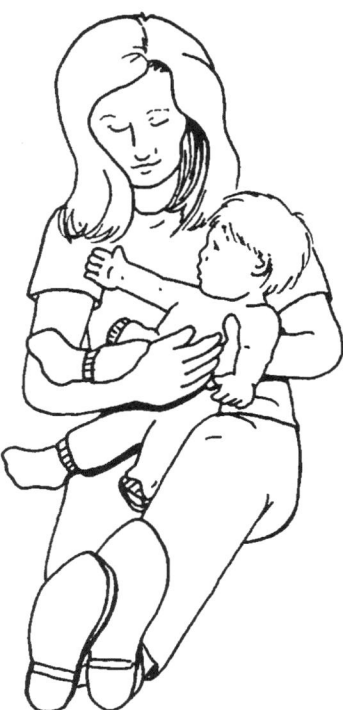

Figure 2b. Shifting the baby's weight toward the hips brings the baby up into sitting sideways on your lap. Allow the baby to help with his head control, if he can.

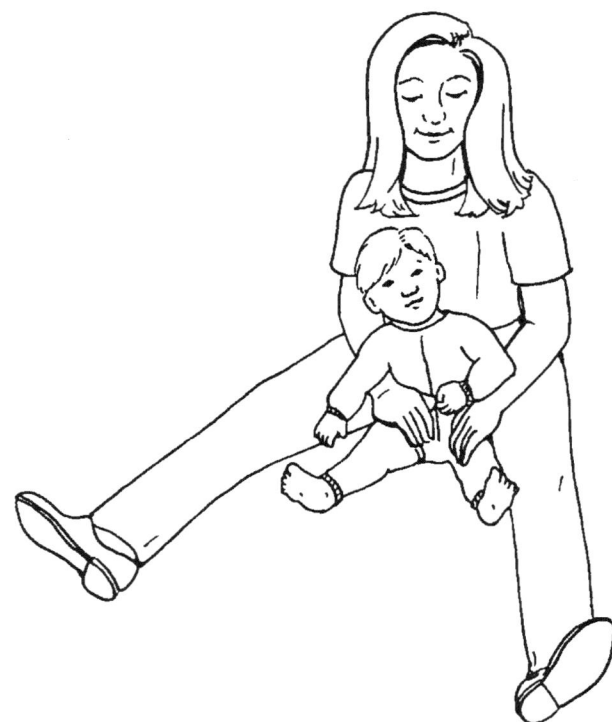

Figure 3. Seat older babies or those who have problems tolerating movement on your lap supported against your body for dressing.

Prepare babies who have problems tolerating movement and/or touch for dressing by giving them deep-pressure input through swaddling or first giving them a hug. You can dress these babies and older infants as they sit on your lap while you sit on the floor so that they are close to the ground. They can sit either supported against your body with their feet supported on the floor or on your lap (Figure 3).

Transitions: Lifting, Putting Down, and Carrying

Is your baby having problems moving or being moved? (Refer to Article 4.2, "Practicing Basic Transitions: Foundations for All Movement Skills").

Infants who are underreactive to movement

Technique No. 1: Babies who are underreactive to movement and have increased or fluctuating muscle tone might have problems initiating movement on their own. They need lifting and carrying techniques that promote head and trunk control. For example, lift the baby by pulling his hips up toward you and flexing his legs toward his tummy. Be careful not to flex the neck. The back of the neck should be flat. Bring his hands to his legs and roll him to side lying with arms and legs together. Wait for him to respond by moving his head in line with his body. Rolling him from side to side or increasing the speed of movement will provide greater input to his movement sense and increase head control. Lift your baby from the surface by supporting his head from behind with your arm underneath, with that same forearm under his armpit and around his chest. Place your other arm between his legs, supporting the trunk on the lower side (Figure 4).

You can carry your baby in this position by keeping the child's body supported against yours or challenging the child by rotating the trunk and head forward and waiting for him to lift his head. Move your baby from side to side while carrying him in this position to provide greater movement input (Figure 5).

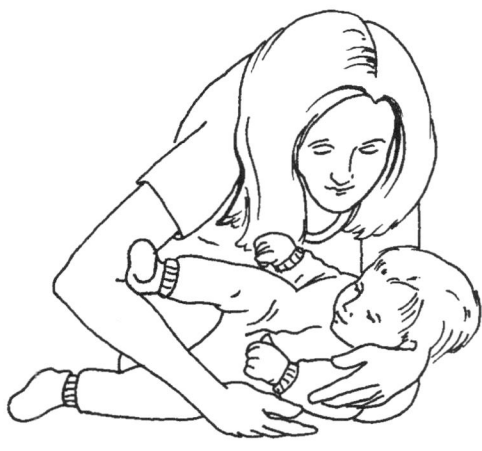

Figure 4. To lift the baby from side lying, place one hand supporting the baby's hand or arm or under the chest. Your other arm goes between the legs, supporting the trunk on the lower side.

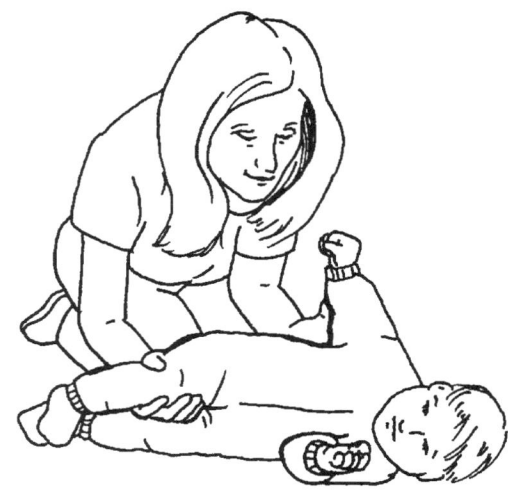

Figure 6a. Move the baby from side lying to lying on the stomach by pulling slightly forward and down on the top leg while keeping the bottom leg straight.

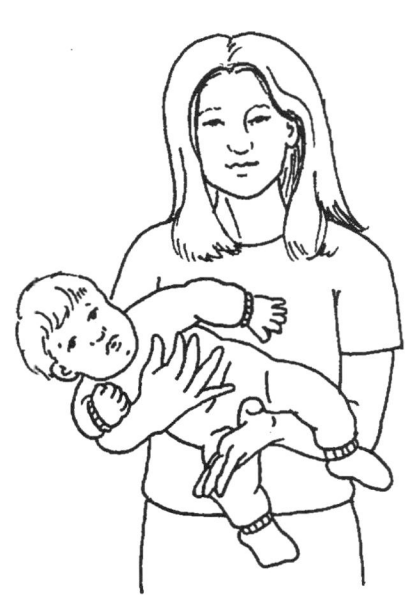

Figure 5. Carry the baby with one arm supporting under the body, coming up across the chest, and the other held between the legs, supporting the lower leg. Support the baby against your body, if needed.

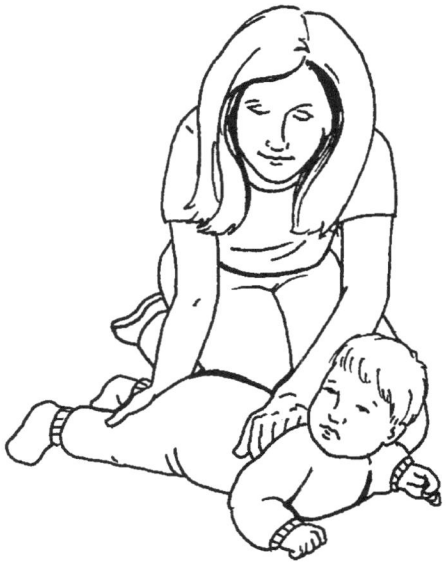

Figure 6b. Roll the baby onto the stomach by moving the upper leg into a straightened position while providing pressure with your forearm onto the child's bottom.

Technique No. 2: If your baby is underresponsive to movement and has low muscle tone but has developed some head control, you can lift him by rolling him from his back to his tummy. First, roll your baby from his back to side lying using the method described in Technique No. 1. Then straighten his lower leg on the side bearing all the child's weight. Move him from side lying to his stomach by slightly pulling forward and down on the top leg, moving it into a straightened position with your forearm on his bottom. Be careful not to pull the leg too firmly. (Don't do this if your baby has dislocated hips.) From this position, place your arm between his legs and your hand on his upper chest as you lift (Figures 6a, 6b, and 6c). Remember, increasing the speed of movement gives more sensory input.

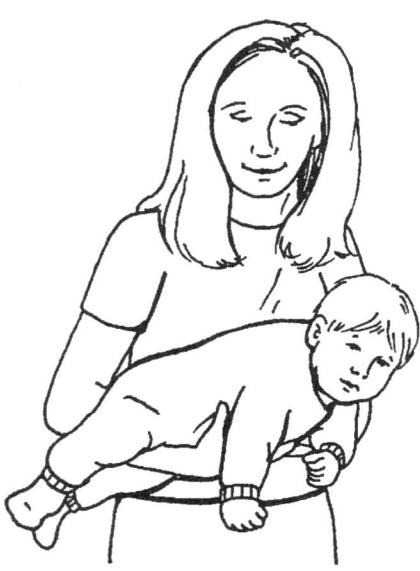

Figure 6c. You can carry your baby by supporting him with your hand between the legs and supporting the upper chest.

Encourage your baby to try to lift his head in response to being lifted upward. You can carry him in this position, providing forward and backward movements to give input to the child's vestibular (movement sense) system. You also can use this carrying position for infants with increased muscle tone who appear underreactive to movement, but not for babies who are overreactive to movement.

Infants who are overreactive to movement

Technique No. 3: You can lift infants with increased, fluctuating, or decreased tone who have difficulties tolerating movement as described in Technique No. 1. Once your baby is side lying, slide him close to your body, place your arm around the back of his neck for support, and use your other hand to keep his legs flexed and together. Lift him from the surface, cradling him close to your body.

Place your baby back on the surface in the same position by cradling him against your body, placing him in side lying, and rolling him on his back, keeping his arms and legs flexed (bent) toward his body. Carry your baby by cradling him, using your arm to support the back of his shoulders and head. For babies with increased tone, you might need to help keep the shoulders forward (Figure 7). Support for the legs will vary. If your baby has increased tone, you can separate his legs by coming between them, slightly flexing the leg closest to you. If your baby has low or fluctuating muscle tone, support the hips and knees together.

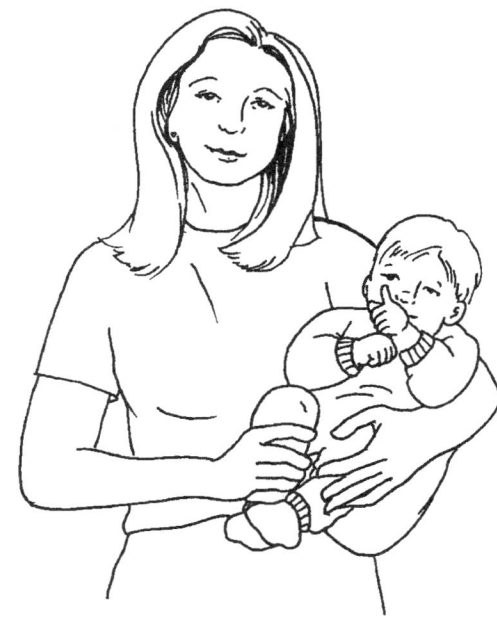

Figure 7. Carry babies with increased tone cradled with your arm behind the shoulders, supporting them forward.

Transition older infants from their back through side lying up to sitting. Lift your baby with his back against your stomach, facing away from you. Keep his legs and arms together in front (Figure 8). You also can carry him in this position, especially if he has low muscle tone. Slowly bounce him up and down while holding him, or sway with your body side to side to provide movement input, always watching for his response.

A carrying alternative that your baby might tolerate more easily is to place his legs straddling your hip while you support his hips and back with your arm, keeping him close to your body. His stomach either can be facing in toward you (Figure 9) or turned forward, depending on his response.

Carrying a younger infant upright in an infant front pack will provide the child with firm pressure all around his body. Provide slow up-and-down movement as you hold the child in the pack.

Handling With Care or Handling Carefully: Sensory Problems in Infants With Cerebral Palsy

Summary

Babies with cerebral palsy can have both sensory and motor difficulties that impact their development and affect interactions with people and objects in their environment. By identifying these specific problems, parents can adjust their handling and caregiving techniques to their babies' individual needs. Parents easily can incorporate sensory and motor adaptations into daily activities of bathing, dressing, playing, lifting, and carrying to improve both movement skills and interaction with their child's world.

For more clarification of Neuro-Developmental Treatment (NDT) theory and how it influences therapy for children, see Article 1.2 by Judith Bierman, titled "Philosophy, Theory, and Principles: The What, Why, and How of NDT."

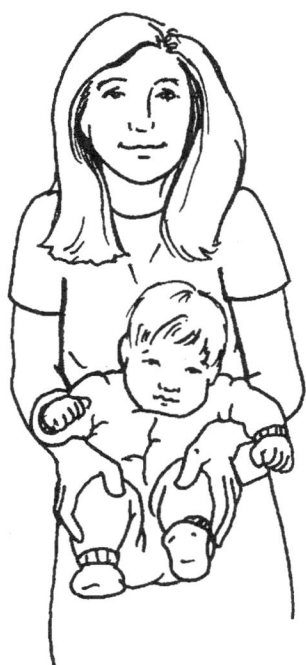

Figure 8. Carry the baby by holding onto the legs, supporting the child against your body. Keep the baby's arms forward and legs together.

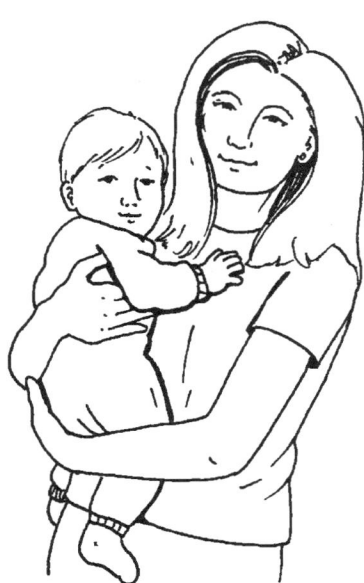

Figure 9. Hold the baby straddling your hip. Support the hips with one arm and the back with the other. Keep the child close to you, facing your body.

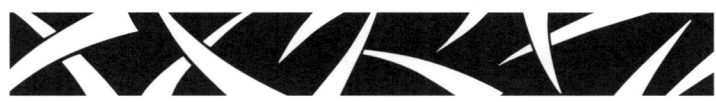

Section 5

Personal Care

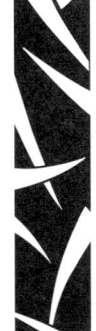

Too Young, Too Soon: Sucking and Swallowing in the Preterm Infant

Robin González, SLP

Feeding is a wonderful way to offer nurture to your baby, and, very importantly, it sets the stage for a lifelong skill. However, parents probably have more anxieties about feeding than any other aspect of the parent-baby relationship.

Feeding is a major area of concern for parents of preterm babies (born too early). What is prematurity? A full-term pregnancy is about 40 weeks, so a premature baby is defined as one who is born before the completion of the 37th week of pregnancy. What does competent feeding mean in terms of the infant's overall health and maturation? First, it is the basis for survival. Next, it provides a way to measure progress, by observing the baby's attentional states (levels of awareness), stamina (strength and endurance) for taking nutrition, and digestive abilities (amount of food and weight gain).

If the feeding process goes smoothly, parents are comforted in knowing that they've met their child's nutritional needs. Successful feeding indicates at least one area of normalcy despite the uncertainties of living with a delicate, tiny, immature system that might be challenged by infection, trauma, lung immaturity, breathing difficulties, or other medical complications.

Feeding not only provides nutrition but also mutually satisfying feeding interactions between infant and caregiver, which help these little babies develop attachment, trust, and communication skills. Furthermore, the feeding relationship can influence the development of a self-identity throughout the first years of life, as well as subsequent learning, problem solving, and language abilities.

On the other hand, when feedings are difficult and the infant-caregiver interaction is interrupted, both infant and caregiver can experience increased stress and frustration. What are the common problems parents experience in feeding a preterm infant?

First, all caregivers need to understand that feeding is a very complex task that involves many different areas of the body, not just the mouth. In addition, feeding is no easy task for babies born early. Because of the shortened amount of time in the womb, preterm infants can have lung immaturity, problems regulating breathing and heart rate, and difficulty coordinating sucking with swallowing and breathing. Sometimes unpleasant experiences with breathing tubes and procedures involving the mouth can affect touch sensations in the throat, mouth, and around the face. Also, some babies are limited in their ability to take in sensory information (light, sound, smell, movement), which interferes with the motor and sensory (or neurobehavioral) skills needed for feeding.

Although bottle or breast feeding often begins for the preterm infant around the 34th week of gestational age, the baby might not have the strength, endurance, or breathing coordination to take all of the needed nutrition by mouth. Alternate feeding methods can help meet these nutritional needs until the baby can manage the whole task independently. Typical alternative feeding methods include providing nutrition through a tiny tube passed from the mouth down the back of the throat to the stomach, or through the nose down to the stomach. This can help the baby's growth so that the infant doesn't have to work too hard and risk sacrificing the development of a pleasurable experience.

Feeding success typically is the last obstacle that the hospitalized infant needs to overcome. It is one of the factors indicating readiness to go home. Often there is a great deal of emphasis placed on the infant and caregiver to complete this task hastily. Starting feedings too soon or pushing feedings (insisting that the baby take consecutive feedings or take every feeding by mouth) before the baby is ready doesn't speed up maturity and guarantee success. Instead, disregard of the infant's individual responses can contribute to prolonged hospitalization and feeding difficulties in the present and future. Feeding success isn't measured by volume alone. It is dependent on the skills that the baby as well as the caregiver bring to the activity!

Ideally, you need to focus on your baby's individual characteristics and feeding-readiness cues and your own understanding of these cues. You need to consider many factors:

- gestational age
- ability to regulate breathing and heart rate
- muscle strength and support of the head and neck
- presence of mouth, throat, and swallowing responses
- ability to arouse spontaneously and show signs of hunger
- ability to tolerate the surroundings (light, noise, and movement)

Frequently, these early communication signals are subtle and difficult to interpret in the preterm population. As a result, the baby's pacifier sucking often is the only cue considered in assessing feeding readiness. In fact, sucking on a pacifier is a completely different skill from sucking that results in food intake. Sucking used for taking in food is called nutritive sucking. It requires much more skill and coordination on the part of the infant because of the complexities involved in sequencing and coordinating breathing and swallowing.

Because each baby brings unique characteristics to the feeding experience and each caregiver brings unique skills to the feeding activity, a primary goal aimed toward achieving a pleasurable feeding experience is to develop understanding and awareness of the communication between the two partners.

Neuro-Developmental Treatment (NDT) Principles

NDT principles can provide a foundation for the following suggestions to improve this communication.

- **NDT Principle:** Development or skill acquisition relies on the body's neural maturation, interaction of its many systems, and its interaction with the environment.

  Activity: Watch for your baby's unique feeding-readiness cues. Identify signals of stress and those that indicate that the child is calm and stable. Take inventory of everything going on during the feeding in order to determine what you might need to add or take away. In other words, adjust your baby's internal and external environments to support the child's current skills.

  Method: Modify temperature, light, noise, and/or activity level as appropriate. Increase or decrease the lights, sounds, movements, or smells to which the baby is exposed during feeding time. Consider the number and types of stimulation presented simultaneously. For example, rocking, talking, and feeding might be too much at the same time. Changing the temperature of the room to warm or cool your baby might help him feed more successfully.

- **NDT Principle:** Normal movement requires good body alignment and support so that the muscles can work most efficiently.

  Activity: Holding your baby while she sucks on a pacifier or takes a bottle

  Method: Provide some support on the outside of the baby's body by swaddling or wrapping her in a blanket so that her legs and arms aren't flailing in space or dangling away from her body. Help the arms tuck toward the body, with hands up near the face. Placing your finger in her hand or offering a small object that fits inside her hand for grasping helps improve sucking. Her hips should be slightly bent at the waist.

  Supporting her head so she has a little bit of a chin tuck also helps her sucking and swallowing. Hold your baby in a more upright position rather than reclined (lying back) to help her coordinate her swallowing muscles. All of this support helps her have better control and decreases her stress, allowing more energy for feeding.

- **NDT Principle:** Mobility depends on supported stability including the automatic, internal rhythms of the body.

  Activity: Sustained nutritive sucking

  Method: The ability of your baby to move his tongue and jaw successfully for sucking and swallowing depends on the support of his body and the support of the nipple, paired with his breathing pattern. A natural way of cueing him to open his mouth for the nipple is to stimulate a rooting response. With your baby well supported, gently stroke on the bottom lip or off to one side of the mouth. You can use a pacifier at first to help the baby get ready to take the nipple on the bottle. If his tongue tip is stuck up against the roof of his mouth, gently massage under his chin in a circular motion to help the tongue find a position that will allow acceptance of the nipple. Avoid forcing the nipple into the baby's mouth. This is an unpleasant experience.

  Once your baby has opened his mouth to accept the nipple, gently place it in a stable position against the roof of his mouth, toward the front, so that you don't set off a gag reaction. It is much easier for the tongue to find the nipple when it is in a stable position. The baby's tongue then can start the movement needed to pull the nipple into the correct place toward the back of the mouth for sucking.

  Watch the baby's sucking and breathing pattern. Both patterns are rhythmic activities like the beating of the heart. Breathing needs to occur regularly. It should be paced at least every three to five sucks. You can accomplish this either by tipping the bottle slightly downward to interrupt the liquid flow or by removing the bottle from the baby's mouth at the right intervals. Babies who are not yet full term (40 weeks) frequently need this pacing to alert them to this breathing/sucking pattern.

  Sometimes, helping the baby pace his breathing can increase the baby's intake of air, so burp the child more often. The rhythm of gently patting the baby's back or slowly rocking the infant's body from side to side should reinforce a slow, rhythmic response. This smooth rhythm helps the baby regulate and calm his internal body as he tries to process all the information coming in from the external world.

- **NDT Principle:** Parents/Family are integral in caring for and nurturing the infant.

  Activity: Enjoyable feeding experiences

  Method: Whether your baby still is hospitalized or has come home, make sure that all professionals working with you support your family's values and beliefs, provide useful information, and build confidence in your ability to recognize your baby's stress and stability cues. Although her communications might seem to be unclear because they don't contain spoken words, she is speaking to you loudly and clearly! You can meet your baby's needs more easily if you understand her language. Identify her strengths, and try to expand those strengths.

Precautions

A feeding problem can get worse if caregivers and professionals misunderstand or don't pay attention to babies' communication signals. You need to share with professionals what you know and observe about your child. At the same time, those professionals need to share information about distinguishing feeding behaviors related to maturity from those that are pathological and cause for concern.

Summary

Feeding is a complex task incorporating many different skills and influenced by factors within the baby as well as in the baby's external environment. These factors are related to each baby's own individual history, experiences, and level of maturation. Feeding is not an exclusive activity involving only the mouth, the nipple, and the formula/breast milk. If you are to establish a successful feeding relationship, you must respect your baby's specific communication signals. These signals begin with basic physiological responses, levels of alertness, attention and energy, coordination of muscle movements, and sensations within the body. As the baby matures and grows older, feeding skills also change and expand, especially during the first year of life. This maturation makes feeding an exciting and dynamic process. New milestones and capabilities are waiting to emerge, always influenced by previous feeding experiences. You have the power to make feeding positive and pleasurable.

For more clarification of Neuro-Developmental Treatment (NDT) theory and how it influences therapy for children, see Article 1.2 by Judith Bierman, titled "Philosophy, Theory, and Principles: The What, Why, and How of NDT."

Help Me Learn to Eat: Sensory Experiences to Facilitate Feeding Skills

Merry M. Meek, M.S., CCC-Sp

Seeing, smelling, and tasting all are extremely important in helping each of us decide what foods we would like to eat. We all know that when we see food, our taste buds are stimulated and more saliva is produced in the mouth. However, we smell food before we see, taste, and then eat it. Many children with feeding problems react (positively or negatively) to the smell of certain foods during its preparation, even before it is presented to them. These children sometimes gag at the taste and texture of the food. Children with neurological disorders have difficulty coordinating the movements needed to process the food in their mouths in order to swallow it.

One of my 9-year-old clients who had never eaten anything by mouth taught me how little she knew about foods. She couldn't associate the smell of a food with a matched picture, name foods, or categorize them although she attended school and had normal intelligence. Her gift to me was that she could talk and tell me the problems she was having as we tried to develop her oral-feeding skills. She preferred smelling the benzoit pads from her 50-plus hospitalizations rather than most foods, which were more unpleasant to her!

Many children cannot eat orally for safety reasons such as aspiration or because extensive hospitalizations and surgeries have required nasogastric or gastrostomy tube feeding. Therefore, they never have had the opportunity to see, smell, or taste foods and liquids or have food come to the mouth by spoon. They haven't experienced an important normal developmental process that prepares every baby for eating: sensory exploration.

While still in the womb, infants not only explore their faces with their hands, they also explore their hands with their faces, that is, with the extremely sensitive mouth area. Experiments with newborns have shown facial changes in response to odors, even without prior feeding experience. Facial expressions also show different responses to sweet, sour, and bitter tastes.

Some normal infants start gagging when shifted from a breast nipple to a bottle nipple, because the tongue posture is different. It also is common for infants to gag when baby foods are introduced at 4 months of age or even later. They learn to adapt to the different smells, tastes, and textures of these foods and to the different shapes of feeding utensils.

When infants start cutting teeth around 5 or 6 months, they want to gnaw on anything they can get to their mouths. Teething biscuits offer a new smell, taste, and texture. Children progress to other soft crackers, cookies, and ground or mashed food as their eating skills develop. Children usually are 3 years or older before they enjoy strongly flavored and textured foods that require a lot of chewing (meat and raw fruits and vegetables, some with skins).

As babies begin to sit safely in a high chair, they also start exploring the foods presented to them by sticking their hands in the bowl, grabbing the spoon, and smearing their faces and the high chair tray. These actions incorporate the appearance, smell, taste, and texture of the food as well as the sensory organization within the hands. This exploration leads to finger feeding and, later, eating with utensils.

We can offer these sensory experiences to children who have been on alternative tube feeding, have resistance to a variety of foods, or who eat a very limited diet and seem to resist, gag, or vomit with the introduction of new foods. The following guidelines can help us provide them with the same sensory experiences as the normally developing child:

- Introduce a good oral-hygiene program so that oral structures are healthy and ready for function.
- Help normalize the child's olfactory responses (reacting to the smell of food) so that the child won't refuse food even before tasting it.
- Help normalize the gustatory responses (reacting to the taste of food) so that the child will begin choosing to eat.
- Encourage hand-to-mouth and toy-to-mouth exploration, which normalizes the child's tactile responses (reacting to the feel of food on areas inside and outside the mouth).
- Encourage hand play with food in preparation for finger feeding.

Neuro-Developmental Treatment (NDT) Principle

We also can help these children improve their eating skills by basing our intervention on an important NDT principle: Good body alignment and seating posture is necessary to maintain an active base of support that allows for efficient use of arms, hands, and mouth.

- **Activity:** Positioning and food suggestions for introducing olfactory exploration (smell)

Method: The seating system should include a table or tray so that the child's arms and hands can rest on the surface. Present food odors such as freshly opened sealed bags of crackers, cookies, canned foods, or flavorings such as vanilla, cinnamon, and lemon. Document the child's preferences. Provide little smelling bags of dried spices for hand play (hand to nose, hand to hand) and even games of rolling the bags back and forth between people. Incorporating smell as a vital part of the therapeutic process can help the child adjust to new and different food items.

- **Activity:** Positioning and food suggestions for introducing tactile exploration (touch)

  Method: Invite the child to be involved in preparation of fruit shakes, fruit and vegetable salads, spaghetti, and cookies with colored sprinkles. Ask the child if you can taste his food. Your obvious enjoyment might motivate the child to take the next step.

- **Activity:** Positioning and food suggestions for introducing gustatory (taste) exploration

  Method: Seating posture should allow the child to bring the hand to the mouth with or without assistance. Offer the child a selection of foods or liquids to taste based on preferences shown when smelling and playing with foods. Some children frequently show aversion to an adult hand coming toward the face because of previous negative experiences with many tubes and medical instruments or force feeding. Therefore, it usually is best to have children taste from their own fingers. Provide crayons and markers, preferably with odors, so that the child can scribble or draw pictures of the foods she has tasted and/or helped make. Look for colorful cereals, different colored lollipops, and thin purees or liquids. The child might want to taste only a few of these, but each attempt at seeing, smelling, tasting, and feeling the texture of food in the hand or mouth is an important step toward eating!

We need to remember that eating generally is considered a pleasurable activity as well as vital to our nutritional survival. Let's make mealtime an enjoyable experience for our children.

For more clarification of Neuro-Developmental Treatment (NDT) theory and how it influences therapy for children, see Article 1.2 by Judith Bierman, titled "Philosophy, Theory, and Principles: The What, Why, and How of NDT."

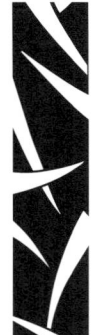

Sit Up at the Dinner Table! Feeding Positioning Tips for Parents

Gay Lloyd Pinder, Ph.D., CCC-SLP

"Sit up straight at the dinner table!" I remember my father often saying this to us as I was growing up. I still can picture myself slouched over my plate and shoveling in the food, then straightening up and looking around at my sisters and brothers as we all sat up straight in response to my father's command. I smile at the memory, but I also remember the effect of the postural change on myself and the interaction of the family. We could see each other and the food on the table. We could talk with each other more effectively.

Children with neuromuscular problems cannot sit up straight easily, but when they have assistance from seating devices, the impact of this command is similar. Sitting with the spine straight and the hips at right angles helps children not only to swallow more easily but also to look around and communicate with those sitting nearby. Sitting with the body symmetrical, head upright, shoulders down, and arms forward helps with self-feeding. Independent feeding can include picking up a cookie, bringing it to the mouth, taking a bite, and putting it down again. It might mean holding a cup, bringing it to the mouth, tipping it to drink, and bringing it back down again without spilling. It might mean holding a spoon or fork to scoop or stab, then bringing it to the mouth and back down again. All of these basic self-feeding skills that are easy for most of us actually are quite complex. They require that the central body be stable before the arms, hands, and mouth (the peripheral parts) can do their jobs.

A basic Neuro-Developmental Treatment (NDT) principle is the idea that postural stability and control are necessary for a person to be able to accomplish tasks such as self-feeding. The primary goal always is for our children to do as much as possible without assistance. For one child, this might be holding the spoon by herself. For another, this might mean keeping his hand on yours as you hold and move the spoon from the bowl to his mouth and back down again. For yet another, this might mean that you hold the spoon while she holds her head up and in the middle, opens her mouth to meet the spoon, then closes her lips around the spoon without biting it.

The first step in a task analysis of feeding is looking at the position of the child's hips, trunk, shoulders, and head. We begin problem solving to make mealtimes work better by deciding which parts of the body need to be stable so that other parts can be as active as possible. Therefore, we don't want to strap children down (or up) so that they can't move. See how complicated eating is when you break it down step by step! The challenge for each child depends on each child's body.

Some children sit in wheelchairs that are designed to provide the stability they need. Other children have special feeding chairs adapted for them to provide that positional foundation. Others sit for mealtimes in their parents' or caregivers' laps because nothing else has worked. This last position is fine for a young baby, but it can interfere with an older child's self-image, decrease opportunities for the child to try to help with feeding, and also limit social interactions with family and friends during mealtimes.

Why is social interaction important during feeding? When children have a difficult time eating, our first concern is nutrition and health issues. Rightly so, parents feel a huge responsibility to be sure that they meet those needs. On the other hand, adults who have severe feeding problems say again and again that the most important part of a meal for them is the social experience, that the food is a necessity but not the fun part. So we must work at positioning to help children make eye contact with others and to see what is happening as they join family or friends at the snack or dinner table. If the feeding process is impossible in that kind of stimulating environment, the child can eat in a quiet place at a different time, then join family and friends at the table for the social experience.

Positioning observations and adjustments should begin at the hips, then move up to the head and down to the toes (Figures 1 and 2, page 102):

- pelvis at 90° (right angle)
- hips neutral so legs are straight and not turned in or out
- active upright trunk (remember my father's command to "Sit up straight!")
- arms level, forward, and rounded, not stiffly extended
- shoulders down and equally straight
- neck elongated so head is not tipped or resting back
- neutral head alignment with head straight and in midline
- feet stable and preferably resting flat on a surface

Sit Up at the Dinner Table! Feeding Positioning Tips for Parents

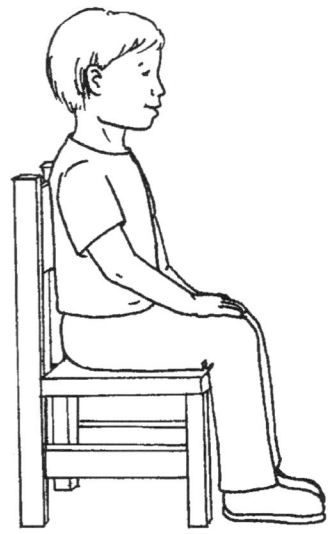

Figure 1. Correct posture.

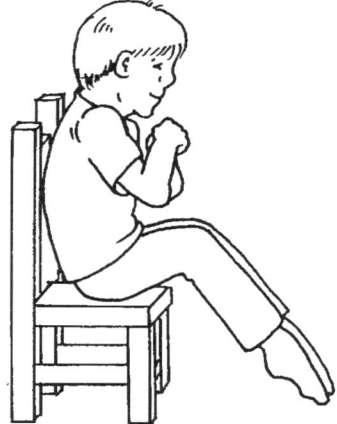

Figure 2. Incorrect posture.

Notice that we started with the hips and then moved up to the head and down to the feet. If the hips are stable with the pelvis at a right angle, the rest of the body all the way up to the head can move into a correct position. Without the hips well positioned, the head and neck can't move into proper alignment. Using these points as a guide, you can become quite creative with ideas for positioning. I have seen a wide range of successful positioning devices from prone standers and wedges to a tractor tire tube! Each of the seats addressed the above points for the individual child's needs.

Normal babies and toddlers sit in high chairs to eat. The high chair puts the young child at eye level with other people who are sitting in chairs, either feeding the child in the kitchen or at the dinner table with the family as they eat together.

Many young children with neuromuscular problems don't have the trunk stability to sit well in a high chair. They might slump to one side or slide under the tray. Without an active trunk or with poor head control, they might hang forward with their head down, which means they can't see and the feeder can't reach their mouth.

We have developed a foam-seat insert (Figure 3) cut with an electric knife from high-density foam for very young children who don't yet have wheelchairs. We custom make these inserts for a specific child and his or her high chair. The goal is to provide additional hip and trunk support so that the child can sit upright in the high chair for feeding, before the child is ready for a more permanent seat such as a wheelchair. These foam inserts have proved to be an excellent and relatively inexpensive way to enable a young child to use a high chair and join the family at the table. Parents or therapists can recut the inserts to allow for the rapid growth that occurs at this age.

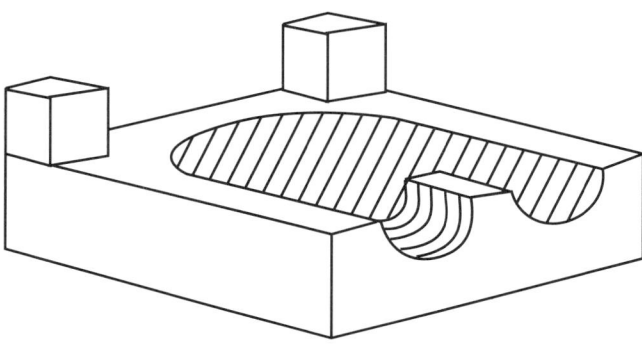

Figure 3. Foam insert.

Other aspects of the feeding environment that influence the child's position are the height and angle of the feeder's position and the position of the spoon or cup. For example, a feeder's face above the child will encourage the child to tip his or her head back and look up to make eye contact for communication. Holding the spoon or cup above the child's eye level also encourages the head to tip back to look at the spoon or cup. Note, however, that many children tend to arch backward or straighten at the hips, and you can trigger this total body response by encouraging the child's head to tip back and the eyes to look up. In order to keep the child's head forward and in midline, the best position is for you to be seated in front and at the child's eye level, holding the spoon and cup either at the child's eye level or below. This way, the child will look forward but not up, and you can control the arching more easily. If the child has low muscle tone and is hanging forward, hold the spoon at eye level but not above, to encourage head lifting but not tipping all the way back.

Sit Up at the Dinner Table! Feeding Positioning Tips for Parents

To summarize, a child's seating position at mealtime will have an influence on eating skills as well as social interaction with others during the meal. Both are important aspects of the success of a mealtime experience. As my father, who used to say, "Sit up straight at the dinner table!" and enjoy yourself!

For more clarification of Neuro-Developmental Treatment (NDT) theory and how it influences therapy for children, see Article 1.2 by Judith Bierman, titled "Philosophy, Theory, and Principles: The What, Why, and How of NDT."

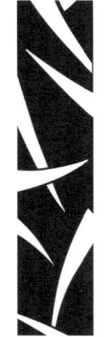

Tube-Feeding Decisions: The What, When, Why, and How

Marybeth Trapani-Hanasewych, M.S., CCC-SLP

Making the Decision to Use a Feeding Tube

The decision to place a feeding tube in a child is at times out of your hands as a parent. It might be so medically necessary that there is no choice. At other times, when the child is still eating orally, you must decide whether the tube should be placed. Here are some key indicators to help make that challenging decision:

1. Consider the amount of time it is taking for each meal and the total time it takes each day to feed the child. If it is taking an hour or more per meal, the value of tube feeding is that it will offer you and your child time to do other, more enjoyable things.

2. Consider the nutritional needs of the child.

    a. Has there been little or no weight gain in the past 6 months?

    b. Are you concerned whenever your child gets ill that he is not getting enough fluids and food to help him get over the illness?

    c. Look at the quantity and quality of hair on your child's head. One of the first signs of good nutrition when your child begins to get foods via a tube is that his hair gets richer in color and thicker in nature.

3. Consider the safety of your child's swallow.

    a. Does she frequently cough, choke, or gag during a feeding?

    b. Is she prone to upper-respiratory infections? Does she tend to get pneumonia in the right lower lobe of the lung? This is where aspiration pneumonia often begins.

    c. Has a modified barium swallow study detected a problem with the child's swallow?

4. Consider the emotional toll on the primary feeder, the child, and the other family members.

The Benefits of Placing a Feeding Tube

1. The type of tube has a major effect on the benefit of the tube. This article refers to a gastrostomy tube or a gastrostomy/jejunum feeding tube.

2. The most significant change that families report is the decrease in life stresses because of the reduced time needed for feeding their children. A bolus feeding takes about 10 minutes. The focus of meals then can be on social interactions and communications between the child and other family members.

3. The child begins to gain weight and grow. Families report how quickly these children grow out of clothes sizes, whereas before the tube, they might have worn the same size of clothing for more than 2 years.

4. The child's hair begins to grow in quantity and quality.

5. The child might become ill less frequently. Attendance in school and/or therapies improves and so do the child's skills. It is a wonderful benefit to be able to watch your child learn and grow.

Making the Decision to Remove the Tube

1. Once a tube is placed, the therapy plan can begin to get the tube removed. The placement of the feeding tube has reduced the medical, growth, emotional, and time-risk factors—now the work begins!

2. Find a professional such as a speech-language pathologist or occupational therapist who has the knowledge base, experience, and interest in helping your child become an oral feeder.

3. Consider the benefits of the tube and try to define therapy objectives you can work toward while the tube is still in place (e.g., the child will be able to enjoy the tastes of food). In some cases, that might be the initial objective in the steps toward tube removal. A possible sequence of objectives toward the goal of feeding-tube removal might look like this:

    a. to enjoy tastes of food at social occasions such as birthday parties.

    b. to enjoy tastes (about 1–6 teaspoons) of food at family meals on a daily basis.

    c. to enjoy and safely be able to eat 2 tablespoons three times per day.

    d. to enjoy and safely be able to eat 4–6 tablespoons three times per day in about 20 minutes. It is at this point that the child's oral-motor skills must improve in order to meet this objective. Also at this point, working with a dietitian will be helpful as you begin to decrease the tube feedings.

4. During this process, consider the following factors as the objectives proceed toward the primary goal of increasing oral feedings and decreasing tube feedings:

   a. It is important to be able to see and appreciate the small gains such as enjoying and safely eating 1 teaspoon of food—with no coughing, choking, or gagging during a feeding trial—and the child enjoying the social interaction at mealtimes.

   b. Be patient because it takes time to make progress and change the oral-motor, sensory, or behavioral components associated with eating that took a long time (until the tube was placed) to be established.

   c. No matter what any professionals tell you regarding the outcome of your child's swallowing or feeding skills, don't stop practicing oral-motor activities. Oral-motor skills do not get better unless they are used.

5. Indicators that the feeding tube can be removed safely:

   a. The child is taking all foods, liquids, and medications orally.

   b. The child has gone through one or two viral illnesses and has maintained or quickly regained weight.

   c. The parents are emotionally ready for the tube to be removed. It is not unusual for families to feel dependent on the tube.

Some families celebrate the tube removal with a graduation party for family and friends. It is a real cause for celebration after the long, emotional road of going to and from a feeding tube.

For further information on this topic, refer to *Feeding and Nutrition for the Child with Special Needs* by Klein and Delaney (Section 9, page 473). See the list of Resources for Parents at the end of this book.

For more clarification of Neuro-Developmental Treatment (NDT) theory and how it influences therapy for children, see Article 1.2 by Judith Bierman, titled "Philosophy, Theory, and Principles: The What, Why, and How of NDT."

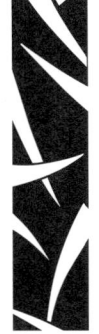

Drooling: Ways to Manage a Difficult Problem

Janet H. Allaire, M.A., CCC-SLP

Drooling is a typical behavior in infancy, especially during periods of teething. By age 4, most children rarely drool. They have learned to manage their saliva by appropriate swallowing and mouth closure. Many children with disabilities, however, still might have saliva falling from their mouths on their faces, clothes, books, toys, and communication systems. Sialorrhea (the medical name for dribbling or drooling) is unsightly, unpleasant smelling, and worrisome. Parents worry that friends, teachers, and other parents will avoid touching this wetness and interact less with the child because of it. Besides being messy, it can cause chapped, rough skin and make problems with fluid intake even more troublesome.

There are four main approaches to handling problems with the drooling: (a) compensatory tactics, (b) surgeries, (c) medications, and (d) therapeutic techniques.

Compensatory Tactics

Compensatory tactics help everyone cope better with drooling although they don't actually reduce the amount of saliva falling from the mouth. For example, special barrier creams applied to the chin prevent the skin from chapping. Some children benefit from special clothing that is super-absorbent and doesn't require changing as often. Deodorant sprays help reduce odor resulting from drooling. Specially designed pillows can prevent children from sleeping in a puddle of saliva.

Surgeries

Surgeries can alleviate drooling for some children. There are two types of surgery. In the first type, surgery interrupts the nerves that stimulate the glands to produce saliva. This surgery is called a tympanic neurectomy and usually is performed by ear, nose, and throat doctors (otolaryngologists). The second type of surgery focuses on the saliva glands and their ducts. The surgeon removes the glands and/or relocates their ducts further back in the mouth and throat. Plastic surgeons usually are the ones to do saliva gland removals or excisions.

Medications

Medications, primarily in the antihistamine category, can reduce drooling but sometimes cause side effects. You'll need to decide whether the side effects are better than the inconvenience of drooling. Some medications, such as glycopyrrolate or Robinul™, have fewer side effects, and doctors prescribe them frequently to reduce drooling. Physicians can provide more information about surgeries and medications.

Therapeutic Techniques

Therapeutic techniques for handling drooling include behavior management and hands-on therapy. Behavior management focuses on a goal regarding drooling. The behavior management program consists of a reward or reinforcer combined with a procedure that will prompt the child to produce the desired behavior. As an example, you might decide that the child could be responsible for wiping his own chin. The child is to wipe his chin every time he hears a timer bell ring. The timer bell rings, the child wipes his chin, and he gets a sticker.

Hands-on therapy might involve a Neuro-Developmental Treatment (NDT) approach, used by physical, occupational, and speech therapists. This approach considers the importance of many body systems working together, including sensory as well as motor processes. Experts believe that the perception of sensation within and around the mouth of a child who drools is different from that of other children. Sensation in the mouth or *mouth sense* drives movement of the tongue, jaw, and throat muscles. In other words, during eating, mouth sense tells us when things are ready to be swallowed and actually cues us to swallow. One of the most effective and natural ways to increase sensory awareness in the mouth is toothbrushing. This daily activity not only alters and improves the mouth sense, improving saliva control, but it also maintains healthy teeth and gums.

Toothbrushing

Position the child near a sink, or hold a small basin under the child's face and mouth during the toothbrushing. Remember that movement patterns for functional activities are most efficient when the body is well aligned, symmetrical, and secure (Figures 1, 2, and 3).

Drooling: Ways to Manage a Difficult Problem

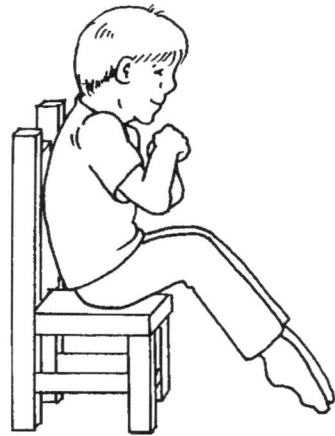 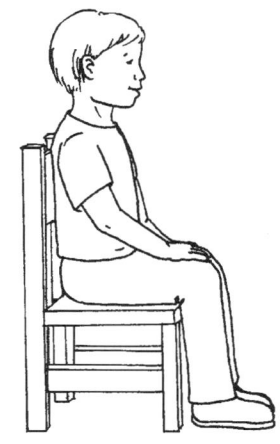

Figure 1. Buttocks should be well back and hips well flexed.

a. Incorrect posture.	b. Correct posture.

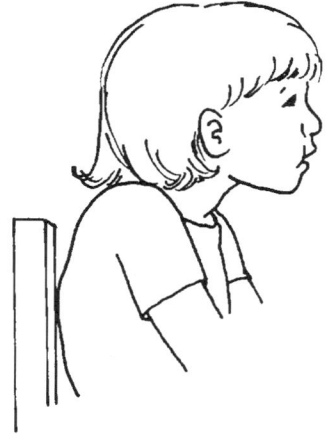 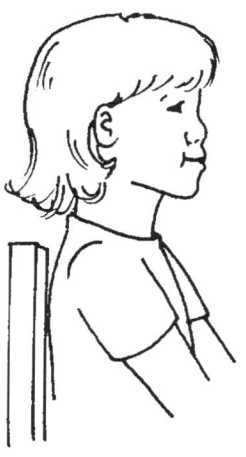

Figure 2. Head should be in midline and forward with chin down.

a. Incorrect posture.	b. Correct posture.

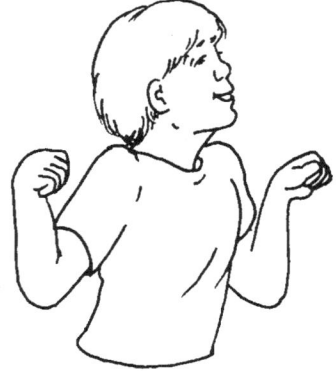 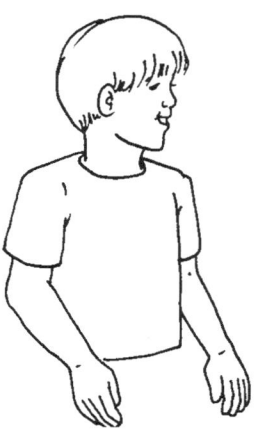

Figure 3. Shoulders and arms should be in forward position.

a. Incorrect posture.	b. Correct posture.

Drooling: Ways to Manage a Difficult Problem

If your child's gums bleed easily, wrap gauze around your finger and use it to rub your child's gums and teeth as an interim step to prepare the gums for a toothbrush later. The toothbrush should be small with soft bristles. You and the child might prefer a battery-powered toothbrush, but the brush should make only small movements and should not startle the child. Toothpaste might not be easy for the child (and you) to manage. An alternative to toothpaste is mouthwash diluted in water. Dipping the toothbrush into diluted mouthwash gives the child the minty taste of toothpaste without the foaming action or slightly gritty mouth sense. Some children prefer baking soda or table salt instead of toothpaste.

Start on the upper teeth on the less involved or affected side of the child's mouth. Think of each tooth as having three sides: the outside, the inside, and the cutting edge. If you provide manual oral control for your child during eating, it is also likely to be beneficial during toothbrushing.

1. Brush the outside of the upper teeth and gums with small, circular motions. It is best to keep in constant contact with the teeth. Stop when you have finished the upper teeth and let the child spit out the excess saliva and/or toothpaste. Teach spitting to children who seem to be having trouble. Using one hand, come underneath the child's chin with your thumb on one cheek and your forefinger on the other. Move your thumb and forefinger forward, gently pinching the cheeks. Bend the child's head toward the sink or basin and say, "Spit." Gradually decrease your manual assistance as the child practices this skill.

2. Brush the outside of the lower teeth in the same manner. Be precise and efficient in your movements. Stop after each side to let the child spit.

3. Begin with the inside of the upper teeth. After completing the inside of the upper teeth, brush the cutting edge of the upper teeth.

4. Brush the inside of the lower teeth, brushing the cutting edge of these teeth last.

5. Brush the tongue one time. Begin at a tolerable point in the middle of the mouth and make one firm stroke to the tip of the tongue. Brush only the front half of the tongue, so as not to make the child gag. If you do gag the child accidentally, don't worry. It might not be fun, but it won't do any harm.

6. Allow the child to spit out the excess saliva or toothpaste. This toothbrushing procedure should take about 2 minutes to complete.

To summarize, the four main approaches to the difficult problem of drooling include (a) compensatory tactics such as creams, deodorants, special clothing, and pillows; (b) surgery on nerves or salivary glands; (c) medications, especially antihistamines; and (d) therapeutic techniques including behavior management and hands-on therapy.

For more clarification of Neuro-Developmental Treatment (NDT) theory and how it influences therapy for children, see Article 1.2 by Judith Bierman, titled "Philosophy, Theory, and Principles: The What, Why, and How of NDT."

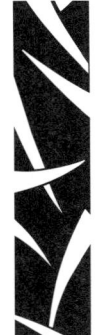

Caring Strokes for Little Folks: Therapeutic Pediatric Massage

Kathy Fleming Drehobl, B.S., OTR/L
Mary Gengler Fuhr, B.S., OTR/L

Touching and holding children is a wonderful way to say, "I love you." Touch is important in determining how children grow, learn, and feel secure. We all know how good a hug from a loving person makes us feel. Touching is good for health! Massage is one of the special ways you can give loving touch to your children. If your child has special needs, massage can provide even more benefits. This article will answer the why, when, what, and how questions about therapeutic pediatric massage. Therapists who use the Neuro-Developmental Treatment (NDT) philosophy believe in a hands-on approach that is consistent with the principles of therapeutic massage. Talk to your child's occupational or physical therapist about your child's specific needs and how you can adapt massage techniques for those needs.

Why Should I Massage My Child?

Massage has a lot of nice health benefits for children. It can help to improve circulation and nutrition of the skin. It reduces pain. It enhances the function of the immune system, which helps protect the body from disease. Best of all, massage provides a fun time for parent and child.

Children with special needs receive even more specific benefits from massage. Massage can improve flexibility in children with high muscle tone or stiffness so that they can move more freely. Massage also can help children with low muscle tone by stimulating more alertness and encouraging reaching and active moving through space. Many parents report that the tummy strokes seem to help with problems of gas and constipation. However, you always should have a physician check out gas and constipation first, to rule out a medical problem. Children who are extremely sensitive to touch sometimes benefit from massage with a deeper pressure. We find that children often will vocalize more during massage, perhaps because the rib cage is expanding more and they can make sounds more easily.

When Should I Massage My Child?

"With my busy schedule, how can I find the time?" When it works into your day! It is best to massage a child when the child is alert. This is the time when your child is most able to communicate and play with you. It's also the time when massage will be the most positive experience for both of you.

However, if your child has a pattern of irritability at certain times of the day, that might be a good time to do a massage for calming. Slow and rhythmical strokes tend to be most relaxing. You also can use massage to wake up your child gently and make the morning routine more pleasant.

- Massage the child's legs at diapering time.
- Massage feet and hands before or after wearing orthotics. Be careful to wipe off excessive oil or lotion before putting on socks.
- Bathing also can be a nice time to massage the back, arms, and tummy. You can use liquid soap and soft-textured bath mitts in the tub. Massage also is fun after bath time with a soft towel and long sweeping strokes followed by a nice rub over the pajamas to help your child relax and fall asleep.
- Massage to the face before feeding might help the child who is sensitive to touch and/or has problems in getting the mouth or jaw in the correct positions. Talk to your feeding therapist about your child's specific needs.
- Massage might help a child become more calm before a medical procedure. Helping your child associate touch with being calm also can be useful in many different parenting situations.

The basic message is, work it into your day. Caring for children is extremely time consuming! Massage is meant to be good for you and your child. Enjoy this special time that gives your child many special benefits and feels good.

What Position Should I Use When Massaging My Child?

Positioning will depend on how much your child likes to move around and the type of muscle tone the child has. For instance, if your child has stiffness, you might want to use pillows or a wedge to help the child bend at the hips and keep the head in the center. Conversely, if your child has low muscle tone, you also might want to use either pillows or a beanbag to bring his or her arms, legs, and head to the center.

Massage on the go might be the solution to stressful situation such as visits to the physician, changes of routine, or when your child is overstimulated. Simple back strokes with a calm voice help your child feel more safe and secure. The association of calming touch from massage could help

Caring Strokes for Little Folks: Therapeutic Pediatric Massage

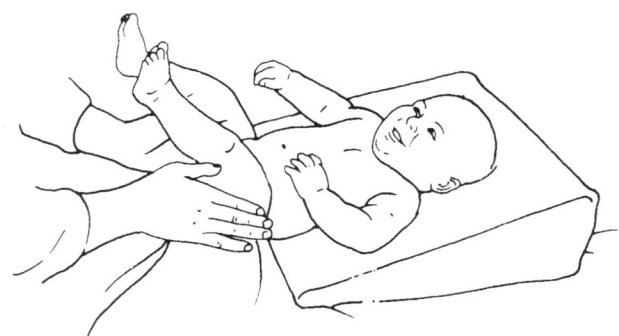

Figure 1.

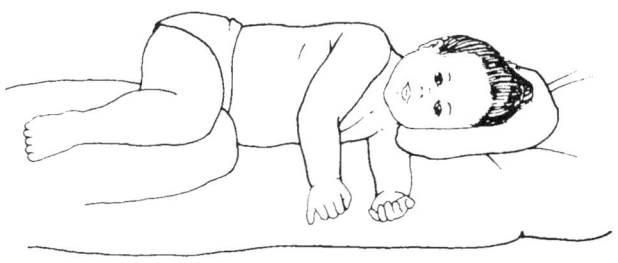

Figure 3.

your child cope with future stressful situations more reliably. If your child doesn't move a great deal, massage probably is best with the child lying face up on a pillow or wedge. You can massage the legs, tummy, arms, chest, and face in this position (see Figure 1). It is important to keep the head in the middle, the arms facing forward, and the legs in a centered position. Rolled-up towels or blankets can help. This position helps your child see you and makes the massage more visually interactive.

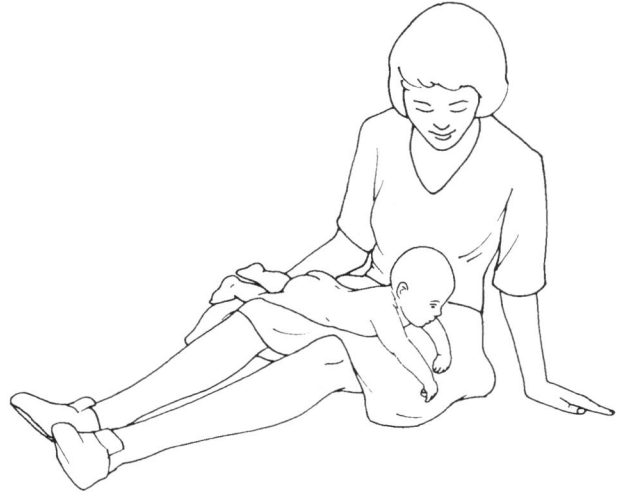

Figure 2.

You can place a small child over your lap when massaging the back (Figure 2). Again, keep the head in the middle with the shoulders forward over your legs. If the child's legs are too far apart, use pillows to bring them together. If the legs are tight together, use a pillow to separate them slightly.

Other positions include side lying with the legs separated (Figure 3), sitting (supported or unsupported), standing, or being held at the shoulder. Your child's therapist can help you determine which positions are best for your child.

What Kind of Oil or Lotion Should I Use?

We have found that natural edible oils and lotions are best for massage because oils and lotions will get on your child's hands and feet and might end up in the child's mouth. Some good choices are almond oil, sesame seed oil, or canola oil (yes, the kind you use for cooking!). Natural lotions are also available at health food stores, bath shops, or even your local grocery. Be sure to read labels to determine what is in these products.

Precautions

- It is important to note that if your child is allergic to nuts, he might be allergic to oils made from those nuts (e.g., almonds/almond oil or peanuts/peanut oil). In this case, *do not* use this particular oil. The safest way to know if a child is allergic to a specific oil is to do a 30-minute skin-patch test. Place a small amount of the oil or lotion onto a small area of skin. Note if there is any redness, and if so, do not use that oil or lotion.
- Ask your dermatologist about massage for a child with acute or chronic skin conditions.
- If your child has allergies or dislikes the oil or lotion, use a favorite blanket or soft hand puppet instead. It works just as well.
- You should *not* use oil on the face because it might get into the child's eyes. Simply wipe your hands with a towel to remove the oil from your hands.
- *Do not* use oil around an open-wound site.

What Signals Will Tell Me What My Child Wants?

Some signs that tell you that your child is ready for a massage might be smiling, reaching for you, or even saying/signing "I want a rub!" Although children usually enjoy massage, there are times when they either need a break or need to discontinue the massage. Initial signs of needing a break include yawning or squirming. Strong signs of a need for the break are crying, whining, or trying to get away by walking, rolling, or crawling. The child literally is telling you, "I've had enough!"

Crying is the only way some children can tell us that something doesn't feel right. We need to respect that either by changing the position or the massage stroke, or by stopping.

How Do I Change the Massage if My Child Doesn't Like a Stroke?

- You can change the massage by stroking more firmly or more lightly. Most children seem to prefer a firm yet gentle pressure; light touch can feel ticklish.
- You also can change the direction of the stroke. For example, some children are very sensitive to strokes that move from the foot to the hip, which goes against the direction of hair growth. You might find that they are more comfortable with stroking that moves from the hip to the foot.
- Your child might prefer to have certain body parts massaged and not others. Most children like having their legs and backs rubbed, so those are good places to start. As you gradually include more areas, you might find that your child eventually enjoys massage in areas that were too sensitive at first.

We all are unique when it comes to the type of touch we like. The name of the game is finding the massage strokes that work for your child. You know your child best and what works best!

How Can I Make the Massage Fun?

Massage should be fun and therapeutic for you and your child. Singing songs about body parts (e.g., "Where is Thumbkin?" and "Head, Shoulders, Knees, and Toes") will be fun and help your child recognize and name body parts. You also can make up your own songs along the way. This is a perfect opportunity for your child to communicate to you what is and is not pleasant. Whether your child communicates with you through speaking, signing, making gestures, or movement, you must listen carefully to what your child is saying. For example, one little girl told us she wanted more leg massage by lifting her leg. No words were spoken, but the message was clear!

What's in It for Me?

Parenting is rewarding but hard work. As you begin to massage your child, you will find yourself relaxing, too. Sometimes, your child will give you a massage in turn.

Is Using Music a Good Idea?

Music can help the child relax or become more alert. Not all children need to become relaxed; some need to be more alert and interactive. Choose the type of music that helps achieve either alertness (more upbeat, stimulating) or relaxation (soft, soothing, rhythmical), whatever your child needs and, of course, what you and your child like.

Some music shops and bookstores carry recordings of streams, ocean waves, and nature sounds. Remember, that for some children who are medically fragile, sound plus touch might be too much stimulation. In this case, use either sound or touch to begin with and gradually add the other.

Medical Concerns

Check with your pediatrician or other specialist before you start massage with a child who is medically fragile or has a fever, a heart or circulatory condition, brittle bones, or other medical conditions. Be sure to explain that therapeutic pediatric massage is not as vigorous as some adult massage. It is very gentle and in most instances safe. However, if your doctor feels that massage strokes could pose a problem, there are some options. Ask your physician these questions:

- Can I safely massage other areas of the body?
- Can I offer just a gentle touch/hand placement without stroking or rubbing?

What About My Other Children?

Brothers and sisters also enjoy receiving a massage! Parents often discover that massage is a nice way to give their other children special time and attention. Sometimes, older siblings can learn to give a massage safely to your child with special needs. This is a great way to create a special bond between your children. Always remember that the person giving the massage benefits as much as the receiver. It is a win-win situation for you and your family!

Do I Need to Do a Full Body Massage Every Time?

A full body massage isn't always necessary. You can choose to focus on one particular area of the body or just use one or two different strokes to several areas. There is no magic number of strokes to do. You'll find yourself getting better at reading your child's cues to determine how much and how long.

How Can I Learn More About Massage for My Child?

Many OTs, PTs, nurses, massage therapists, and special educators have massaged children with special needs. They can teach you specific techniques. A number of great books and videotapes also are available. But remember that your child will be your best teacher!

How Do I Get Started?

You will want to have a supply of towels, small toys, pillows, a favorite blanket, music, and a fresh diaper (if needed). You can warm the oil by placing the bottle in a cup of warm water (out of the reach of your child). Make sure the room is warm because your child will be wearing only a diaper, bathing suit, or underpants. You can warm towels or blankets by placing them in the dryer for a few minutes. Remove your jewelry so that you don't scratch your child. Most importantly, relax before you start. You might wish to take a few deep breaths, shake out your arms, imagine a peaceful place, or whatever else helps you to relax and enjoy this special time with your child.

What Strokes Should I Use to Start?

The following strokes have been well accepted by most children. Naturally, each child will have a preference and will give you cues to follow. Use your palms or the pads of your fingers, being careful not to dig in with your fingertips or fingernails.

Legs

- Indian Milking: Use long strokes, alternating your hands, to glide down the leg from your child's hip to the ankle or foot.
- Swedish Milking: Using long strokes, glide from ankle to hip, then return from hip to ankle using a somewhat lighter pressure.

Stomach

First, place your hand on your child's stomach with gentle pressure. Wait while your child gets used to your touch. Then move your hand slowly in a clockwise circle, staying well below the ribs.

Chest

Place your hands in the center of your child's chest, just below the collarbone. Slowly move each hand out to the side. Continue to move your hands down over the ribs and then move them back to the starting position.

Arms

Start with both hands in the center of your child's chest. Glide each hand out (at the same time) to the shoulder and down the arms.

Back

Cup your hand slightly and glide it down the center of the back, moving from the head or neck to your child's bottom. The cupping allows you to give gentle pressure to the muscles on the side of the spine without putting pressure on the spine itself.

Face

Do not add oil. Place the pads of your fingers in the center of your child's forehead. Move your fingers gently and slowly out across the forehead, down the temples, then inward on the cheeks and toward the mouth.

Important! Your child should drink plenty of water and fluids afterward. And remember to relax and enjoy the massage experience. You both deserve it!

Artwork copyright © 1991 by Kathy Fleming Drehobl and Mary Gengler Fuhr. *Pediatric Massage for the Child with Special Needs*, 0761643095 (Video), 0761647031 (Manual). Reprinted with permission.

Article 4.9, "Making Movement Easier Through Touch," contains additional information on touch.

For more clarification of Neuro-Developmental Treatment (NDT) theory and how it influences therapy for children, see Article 1.2 by Judith Bierman, titled "Philosophy, Theory, and Principles: The What, Why, and How of NDT."

Leaning and Lifting: Practical Use of Weight Shifts for Adolescents and Adults

Laura Vogtle, Ph.D., OTR/L

There are many reasons people with cerebral palsy have trouble moving. One reason is that almost all individuals with cerebral palsy have problems moving weight off a part of the body, unloading an arm or a leg, for instance, so that it can be moved. Think about what you do when you walk. You lift one foot and put it in front of the other. Try taking a step without moving your weight off that foot. What happens? Can you move the foot at all? Now you can understand why these weight shifts are so important and why not being able to shift weight causes problems for those with disabilities.

Everyday activities such as getting on and off the toilet or in and out of the bathtub can be big challenges. Getting dressed and undressed also is difficult if a person can't lift a leg to pull pants up or down. Fear is a big factor, especially as children grow into adolescence and adulthood. Many are afraid that they will fall if they shift their weight. This kind of fear can make lifting or moving a child or adult with cerebral palsy even harder, and yet weight shifts are necessary to make care easier for parents and other caregivers.

Young babies use certain methods to shift weight at first. They lean toward the part they want to move. This makes it harder to get anywhere because their weight is still on the arm or leg they're trying to move. As babies get older, they learn to move body parts by first leaning away from them to take the weight off.

Children with cerebral palsy try to move in the same immature ways as do young babies. They don't learn to change the direction of their weight shifts. Therefore, it's hard for them to move their arms, legs, or bodies, or even to let other people help them move from one place to another. Most children with cerebral palsy try to move using their muscle stiffness (spasticity) instead of weight shifts. This stiffness can be very strong and unfortunately pushes in the opposite direction from that desired.

When you and I change our body position, we lean in one of three directions: forward/backward, side to side, or diagonally (when reaching for the left foot with the right hand, for example). People who cannot move by themselves can make tasks easier by leaning in the correct direction when someone else is helping them with dressing, bathing, or toileting. If the person (child or adult) is unable to begin the leaning movement, the caregiver needs to select the direction that will make the job easier and assist the individual to lean in that direction.

An important part of Neuro-Developmental Treatment (NDT) is learning to use weight shifts appropriately to facilitate more active and effective movement. This NDT principle will be illustrated with examples of methods to assist people with cerebral palsy in bathing, toileting, and dressing activities. Weight shifts also are important for caregivers to protect their own bodies during the process.

Dressing/Undressing

- **Position:** Lying down on the bed (This position often is used to dress people who cannot sit by themselves.)

   Direction of the weight shift: side to side

   Method: Sit on the bed or on a chair or stool beside the bed, not bending over at the waist. Raise the head of the bed, if necessary. Ask the person being dressed to move the arms and legs, or move them yourself. For example, if a leg is lying on the bed, lift it to pull the pants on rather than trying to pull the pants up with the person's leg resting on the mattress. Roll the person to one side, leaving one arm and leg free of the mattress during dressing or undressing. Then roll the individual to the other side.

- **Position:** Sitting on the bed/chair to put on shirts and dresses

   Direction of the weight shift: forward

   Method: Sit on a chair by the bed or in front of the wheelchair. Slip the clothing on over the person's head. Next, ask or help the person lean forward against your shoulder. You then can pull the clothing down the back and over the arms comfortably. Be sure the person being dressed is bending at the hips as much as possible when leaning forward.

- **Position:** Sitting on the bed/chair to put on pants

   Direction of the weight shift: forward

   Method 1: Put the pants on over the feet and pull up as far as possible while the person sits in the wheelchair. Be sure to lift the legs to get the pants up to the hips. Then bend the person forward at the hips and support the knees (Figure 1a). Stand the person up and, with the person's body leaning against yours, pull the pants up (Figure 1b). Lean the person forward again to sit down so that you can control the speed of the movement.

Leaning and Lifting: Practical Use of Weight Shifts for Adolescents and Adults

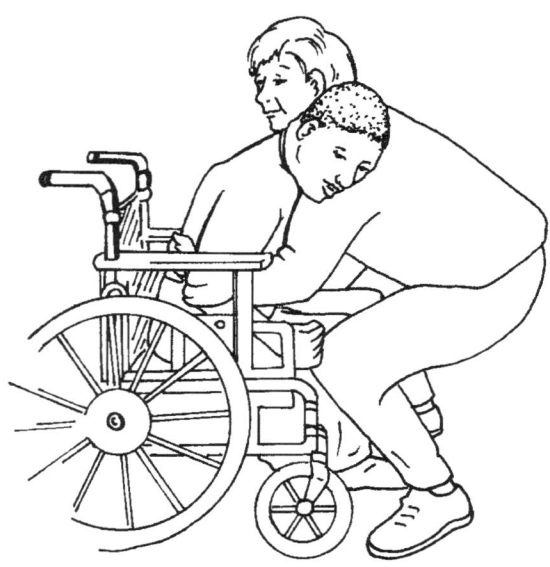

Figure 1a. Bend the person forward as far as possible at the hip.

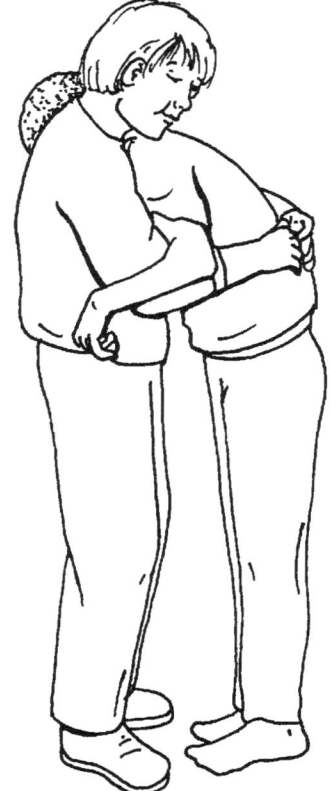

Figure 1b. Pull pants up.

Method 2: Pull the pants up to the hips as described through Figure 1b. Lean the person to one side, making sure that the weight is shifted off the hip being dressed. Figure 2 shows how to be sure the body weight is off one hip. Put one hand under the arm of the person being dressed, and push the weight to the opposite side. Try to lift the leg to see if you can move it freely. Pull the pants up as far as you can, then lean the person to the other side and pull the pants up. It might take several leans to get the pants up high enough. During the side-to-side leans, be sure to keep the person leaning forward at the same time.

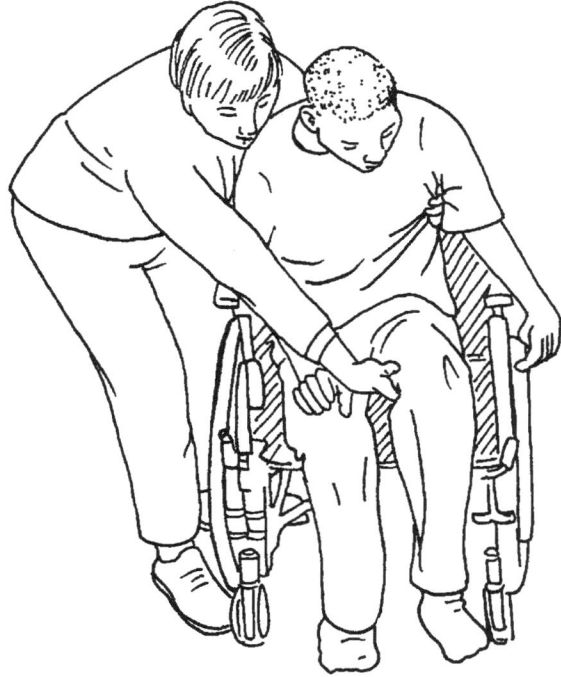

Figure 2. Be sure body weight is off one hip.

Bathing

One of the biggest problems in bathing, in addition to the lifting, is reaching all the body parts. This particularly is true when a large person is lying in a bath chair. You can use the methods described here in both reclining bath chairs and those that hold the bather upright.

Washing the back

Direction of the weight shift: (1) forward, (2) diagonal, (3) side to side

Method 1: Lean the person forward in the tub seat. Use your hand to push gently on the low back if necessary. Put your arm under both the bather's arms as a support. Be sure the bather is bent at the hips. Keeping your arm under the bather's arms, wash the back and rinse. If the forward weight shift is done properly, you should be able to reach to the buttocks.

Method 2: This method requires more movement on the part of the caregiver. Standing at the side of the bather, reach across the front of the person's body to the opposite shoulder. Grasp the shoulder and arm and bring it across the body, with a diagonal weight shift. Change your grasp so that you can hold the bather in this rotated position and wash the half of the back that you can reach. Switch sides and repeat the process on the other side.

Washing the buttocks and genitals

Method 1: Sitting beside the bather, push gently sideways so that the bather's body weight moves all the way to the far hip. Gently lift up the thigh nearest you, and pull it forward. This frees the leg nearest you so that you can reach the buttocks and genital area on one side. Repeat on the opposite side to get the entire area.

Method 2: Bend the person forward at the hips. From the back, put your arm around the bather's waist, keeping your arm as low as possible. From this position, pull gently forward and lift the bather's bottom at the same time. Wash the area, then move the person down and back gently. If you are washing the person in the bathtub, you always should be sitting to prevent bending at the waist or lifting with the back. Both practices can cause injury to the caregiver.

Toileting

The hardest parts of toileting are getting clothing up and down and bowel hygiene.

Direction of weight shift: (1) forward, (2) side to side, and (3) diagonal

Method 1: It usually is easier to get clothing down before the person is on the toilet. You can use a forward weight shift to a stand to pull the clothing over the hips, or you can use Method 1 described previously for buttocks and genitals with side to side weight shifts, in order to get the pants down or up while the person is sitting in the chair. If the toilet is next to a wall, preferably one with a grab bar, lean the person toward the wall and lift the leg farthest from the wall. This should shift the weight onto the hip farthest from you and allow you to bring the free leg slightly forward with a diagonal weight shift so that you can wipe. Do this in front or to the side of the person.

Method 2: If there is no wall next to the toilet, try sitting next to the person to get a forward lean with your arm under both the person's arms. Do a forward weight shift to lift the person's bottom off the toilet seat so that you can wipe. This job will be easier if the person's feet can touch the floor and bear weight.

Summary

Most caregivers get used to doing things in certain ways that work well. The problem is, their bodies get older and less strong, and the children get bigger and heavier. Caregivers need to stop and take a look at how they manage, especially during their children's growing spurts. Readjusting the techniques you use can be a challenge but it can prevent injuries and pain.

Using weight shifts properly can make a job far easier. Pushing and pulling the total body weight, even that of a small adult, to carry out routine care is hard work. By going slowly, sitting instead of standing, and being sure the hips move during the weight shifts, you can make daily living tasks such as dressing, bathing, and toileting simpler and more comfortable for all concerned.

For more clarification of Neuro-Developmental Treatment (NDT) theory and how it influences therapy for children, see Article 1.2 by Judith Bierman, titled "Philosophy, Theory, and Principles: The What, Why, and How of NDT."

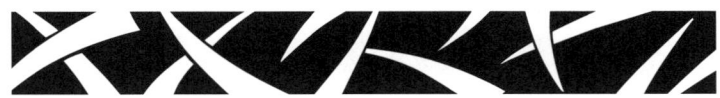

Section 6

Play and Recreation

Play or Therapy? Make Time for Both!

Anita Bundy, Sc.D., OTR, FAOTA

Children with disabilities and their parents confront an important problem every day—the play-versus-therapy debate. When is it time for play and when is it time for therapy? The reasons for this problem are numerous, but they stem from two simple facts. First, there are only so many hours in a day. And second, there is a pervasive belief in American society that playing is a waste of time. This article offers a much more positive view of play and its benefits. It examines the problem in more detail, casts play in a new light, and offers some simple ways to promote play.

Almost 20 years ago, Sonia Diamond, a woman with athetoid cerebral palsy, wrote a compelling book chapter called, "Growing Up With Parents of a Handicapped Child." In her chapter, Diamond grappled with the problem of play versus therapy. She said:

> "*Something happens in a parent when relating to his disabled child;* he forgets that they're a kid first [emphasis added]. *I used to think about that a lot when I was a kid. I would be off in a euphoric state, drawing or coloring or cutting out paper dolls, and as often as not, the activity would be turned into an occupational therapy session. 'You're not holding the scissors right.' 'Sit up straight so your curvature doesn't get worse.' That era was ended when I finally let loose a long and exhaustive tirade. 'I'm just a kid! You can't therapize me all the time! I get enough therapy in school every day! I don't think about my handicap all the time like you do!*'"(Diamond, 1981)

Parents (and therapists too!) often want to combine play with therapy, but that can be extremely difficult. Play and therapy can run at cross purposes. The goal of therapy often is to perform a skill in a particular way. The goal of play is the enjoyment of play itself. As Diamond points out, too much emphasis on "therapizing" can ruin a good play session.

Being a child with a disability is a full-time job. Not only must that child do everything her able-bodied peers do, things that easily fill a day, but she also has to learn to do them right. To move normally, a child with a disability must expend enormous amounts of precious time and energy. What about playing? That's important too. Yes, but not as important as learning to walk and talk and use a pincer grasp. Or is it?

Children are not the only ones whose play is interrupted by therapy. Although adults might prefer the terms *leisure* or *recreation*, play is not only for children. Adults also experience its benefits. To be the parent of a child with disabilities is more than a full-time job. Not only must these parents orchestrate and conduct all the events of their own lives, but they also must plan and coordinate those of their children and additionally all the extra needs of the child with a disability. There is work and housework, meals, crises, and, yes therapy. When is there time to play, with or without the children?

Why play? What are the benefits of play? Clearly, it's hard to find time in busy lives for anything considered unnecessary, and the work ethic historically pervasive in American society suggests that play is unnecessary. If we have free time, should we not use it to better ourselves? It would take a pretty compelling argument to convince most parents that there are many times when play is more important than therapy.

However, current theoretical principles of the Neuro-Developmental Treatment (NDT) approach suggest ways for therapists to provide caregivers with daily activities that integrate therapy into functional skills rather than a set of separate exercises. These principles also recognize that the child is more important than the body parts and that the child functions within the family environment as an individual with a unique personality.

I have been a therapist for 25 years and have been studying play seriously for about half of that time. The more I study, the more I believe that play is one of the most valuable activities in which humans engage. Let me share some of the evidence with you.

There is ample research telling us that children develop motor, social, and cognitive skills in play. However, skill development is somewhat *inadvertent*. Children don't play with the idea of developing skills. It just happens. When a child truly is motivated, as he is in play, he might repeat an activity hundreds of times. Skills and knowledge are developed through repetition. Because play is so highly motivating, it is one of the most effective ways to learn.

Skill development is a good reason to encourage children with disabilities to play. But it is only one of many even more important reasons—those derived from the characteristics of play itself.

First, to succeed in an able-bodied world, children with disabilities need to be adaptable. There are so many physical and social barriers in life that require alternate solutions. There is no right way to play! When we encourage children to play, they learn to be adaptable.

Second, we tell others that we are playing by giving them cues that our actions are not serious. We use a silly voice, or dress up, or exaggerate our words and actions. Similarly, we know when another person is playing because of the cues he gives. The ability to give and respond to cues is useful in many daily situations. For example, we know how to behave in church and school and on the job by reading cues. The thing about play that makes cues easy to learn is that play cues are exaggerated. Because many children with disabilities have little knowledge of their bodies, giving cues and reading them might not come naturally. They need to play with others to learn this important social ability.

Finally, but no less important, as children give cues, they express who they are as individuals. When we respond to those cues, children get the message that we care about what they think and want. There is nothing sadder than a passive, easy, good child who never expresses her needs or desires and whose true self is a mystery to herself, her family, and the world. The best way to help a child become a whole person is to notice and promote those activities in which she becomes totally involved and experiences joy. To give a child permission to play is to give her permission to celebrate her unique life. What better reason could there be?

Playing With Your Child

- Set aside a little time as often as you can for doing things you and your child both enjoy. Make it a time when you tend to be less productive anyway. (I try to play early in the morning because it's not a good time for me to do things that require a lot of thought or energy.)
- Play time is for play. Don't correct your child's posture or movement during that time. Don't think of this as a time to teach.
- Whatever you're doing, do it together. Don't be afraid to get down on the floor, get dirty, or do things you'd be embarrassed to have the neighbors see.
- Match the activity to the time of day and vice versa. If the best time to play is right before bed, roughhousing might not be the best activity. But if roughhousing is your child's favorite play activity, try to find a good time for it.
- Follow your child's lead as much as possible.
- A lot of very good play happens in the context of activities such as housework or yard work.
- Children delight in doing things they see as mischief. Help them. Join them.

Promoting Your Child's Play

- Be unobtrusive. Let the child solve his own problems as much as possible. Don't worry about whether you're meeting therapy goals.
- Make places safe for play by minimizing the consequences of a fall rather than preventing your child from trying her skills. There are many ways to keep children safe. Rules are only one way.
- Avoid power struggles. Consider why you made the rule. Is that one really necessary?
- Explain your child's needs to a responsible peer or nonfamily member. Then let the two of them play together without interruption from you.
- The best toys are ones that have no predetermined outcome—sand, water, mud, finger paints, etc.

Summary

Therapy is important. Developing skills, maintaining the integrity of joints, and becoming independent are important. But independence takes many forms, and there are only so many hours in a day. If I had to choose, I would sooner demonstrate my independence through my adaptability and my wholeness as a person than through my ability to move or talk or perform all my self-care tasks independently. I gain independence through play.

I received the following story by e-mail not long ago. It speaks to the importance of spending our time wisely.

Imagine that there is a bank account that credits your account each morning with $86,400. It carries no balance from day to day and every evening cancels whatever part of the amount you failed to use during the day. What would you do? Draw out every cent, of course!

Actually, everyone has such a bank. Its name is time. It carries over no balance. It allows no overdraft. Each day it opens a new account for you. Each night it burns the remains of the day. If you fail to use the day's deposits, the loss is yours. There is no going back. There is no drawing against tomorrow.

Live in the present on today's deposits. Invest so as to get from it the utmost in health, happiness, and success! The clock is ticking away. Make the most of today. Treasure every moment you have. And treasure it more because you shared it with someone special, special enough to spend your time. And remember, that time waits for no one.

Diamond, S. (1981). Growing up with parnets of a handicapped child: A handicapped person's perspective. I J. L. Paul (Ed.), *Understanding and working with parents of children with special needs*, (pp. 23–50). New York: Holt, Reinhart & Winston.

For more clarification of Neuro-Developmental Treatment (NDT) theory and how it influences therapy for children, see Article 1.2 by Judith Bierman, titled "Philosophy, Theory, and Principles: The What, Why, and How of NDT."

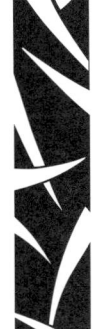

Why Children Love to Play: The Importance of Intrinsic Motivation

Erna I. Blanche, Ph.D., OTR

Children love to play. They like to play with toys. They enjoy moving, running, climbing, and engaging in sports. They like exploring new objects and surroundings. They also enjoy mastering a new skill.

One important characteristic of free play is that it is motivated intrinsically, which means the child's pleasure and satisfaction come from performing the activity, not from an external event. In play, the child exercises intrinsic motivation by choosing to engage in an activity rather than engaging in an activity because of external pressures or reinforcements and/or the approval of others.

Children with physical disabilities have fewer opportunities to play freely and decide their own actions. Sometimes their physical or cognitive limitations interfere with their ability to initiate and enjoy play. Often, therapeutic and educational demands prevent them from having extra time to engage in free play.

During therapy sessions, a child's motivation often is significantly different from the therapist's. The therapist's purpose depends on the treatment goals that are designed to increase functional performance. The child's purpose usually is to enjoy the present activity, not to achieve a future functional goal. Consequently, in order to get a child to perform a specific task, it is important to tap into that particular child's intrinsic motivation. In addition, providing the opportunity for the child to exercise intrinsic motivation can increase the likelihood that the child will practice the movement learned during the treatment session.

All adults (parents, therapists, and teachers) have the responsibility to foster intrinsic motivation in our children as much as we foster self-help, sensory-motor, and academic skills. We can do this by analyzing children's play preferences and thus their intrinsic motivation. For example, a child watching a movie or exploring new surroundings might be motivated by novelty. A child building a tower or putting a puzzle together might be motivated by the pleasure of mastering a skill she has practiced until it is perfect. A child drawing a picture might be motivated by the enjoyment of creating something new and different. A child swinging or twirling might be motivated by the enjoyment of increased sensory stimulation. Hence, the intrinsic motivation to perform a task can be inspired by exploration, mastery, creation, and/or increased sensory awareness.

Your child's therapist might be using Neuro-Developmental Treatment (NDT) principles to plan the treatment, which will help achieve functional goals. NDT treatment principles focus on the production of active movements. Active movements are easier to facilitate when a child is intrinsically motivated to perform a task. Therefore, discovering the child's source of pleasure while engaging in intrinsically motivated activities is a pivotal key to effective treatment.

Therapists try to tap into the child's motivation in order to master a task during treatment. Sometimes, however, the task that the therapist chooses for the child is not the task that the child would like to master. The following examples show how to link types of intrinsic motivation to NDT principles.

For example, a 2-year-old boy with spastic diplegia was motivated to eat by himself. However, every time he took the food to his mouth, flexion in the upper extremities and upper trunk increased. The therapist was afraid that he would eventually develop contractures in this position if he continued using this flexor pattern. Instead of preventing him from performing this activity and hence decreasing his motivation to act on the environment, the therapist solved this dilemma by providing the child with adaptations that allowed him to use the spoon independently and maintain adequate trunk alignment. The boy enjoyed the sense of control he had over the task. This increased sense of control and mastery over the environment then carried over to other treatment activities.

The pleasure of creation is obvious in most preschoolers. However, once they enter a structured academic environment, they are expected to comply with the demands of a structured educational program, and they have little time for free creativity. The therapist can provide an outlet for creativity by preparing an environment that encourages the child to be free to develop his or her imagination.

For example, a 6-year-old girl with spastic diplegia liked to paint. During the occupational therapy session, the therapist placed the child in front of a large piece of paper that encouraged her to elevate her arms to shoulder level. The therapist used the activity to facilitate trunk alignment, shoulder movements, and hand skills. The therapist didn't require the child's painting to look like something real, but instead encouraged the child to express her imagination and intrinsic motivation through her art creation.

Novelty also can serve to facilitate active movement and exploration. When a 2-year-old girl with ataxia was learning to walk, the therapist offered her the opportunity to move up and down the treatment room to a pre-established place. The child showed little interest in standing and even less in ambulating. At the end of the session, however, she was eager to walk to the candy store on the way to the car. The therapist incorporated the child's interest in going out and enjoying novel situations by treating the little girl in different surroundings. One of the activities incorporated into the treatment session facilitated ambulation outside the treatment area. The therapist asked her to deliver papers to other offices or to walk to the cabinets to see what was inside. Each treatment session became an adventure of going somewhere that was mutually decided by the therapist and the child when she first arrived for therapy. The sense of adventure incorporated into the session provided the child with the pleasure of enjoying novel experiences and hence active participation in treatment.

A 5-year-old boy with hemiplegia moved slowly and laboriously. During treatment sessions, he took a long time to perform most movements and, outside of the therapy room, usually required adult intervention to engage in play and self-care tasks. Once, during her conversation with the mother at the end of a treatment session, the therapist noticed that the boy repeatedly threw himself backward on some pillows. He appeared to enjoy this game and became animated doing it. She decided to increase the sensory experience of movement during treatment sessions by asking the child to climb up a ramp and then fall on the pillows. During the climbing phase of the activity, the therapist facilitated transfer of weight to the more involved lower extremity. During the preparation for the falling phase, the child had to reposition his body actively to prepare for the fall, so the therapist facilitated trunk rotation during those transitional movements. The boy enjoyed the activity and repeated it several times, providing an opportunity to address most of his treatment goals focusing on active movement.

The therapists treating these children used the children's intrinsic motivation to participate in treatment activities—mastering a task, the freedom to be creative, the adventure of novelty, and the increased sensory awareness created by an activity. These examples illustrate how tapping into children's motivation to move helps the children reach their treatment goals and provides opportunities for them to exercise a sense of control over their own world.

Parents also can incorporate their children's intrinsic motivation into the daily routine. For example, you can give children choices of what to do, what to wear, and/or what to eat as often as the routine allows it. Create opportunities for enjoying free play with unstructured materials as much as possible. Unstructured materials such as finger paint or play dough allow the child to express creativity. Try incorporating activities that require making small projects such as simple crafts or cooking. These activities can give children a sense of mastery and accomplishment that they later will use in their daily routines.

Other activities you can incorporate into daily routines include outings to movies, plays, or new surroundings. Exposing children to novel situations increases their repertoire of possible child-environment interactions and enriches their memory banks for future transactions. By incorporating activities that are intrinsically motivated and provide a sense of enjoyment, you are advocating for your child's right to express him- or herself as a unique person. What more important gift can an adult bequeath to a child?

For more clarification of Neuro-Developmental Treatment (NDT) theory and how it influences therapy for children, see Article 1.2 by Judith Bierman, titled "Philosophy, Theory, and Principles: The What, Why, and How of NDT."

Vision: Must It Stand Alone?

Rhoda P. Erhardt, M.S., OTR, FAOTA

Parents of children with cerebral palsy and other movement disorders often are aware, even during the first year, that something is wrong with their child's eyes. Parents later tell therapists, "His eyes weren't always straight, especially when he was tired." "She didn't always notice me when I was across the room." "He wasn't interested in books and pictures." "She seemed to ignore everything on one side of her body." "He never watched his hands."

Yet, eye doctors often tell parents that their child is too young to test or, if tested, that the eyes are fine, with normal acuity (ability to focus). However, new techniques allow better testing of infants and young children, and parents have a right to seek another opinion.

It is important to remember that visual acuity is only one component of the visual process. The ability to move the eyeballs quickly and accurately to find or localize an object somewhere in the environment is another crucial component, and the six eye muscles doing that are part of the whole body's neuromuscular system. Dr. Arnold Gesell is well known for his research in child development at Yale University more than 40 years ago. But not many people know that he was especially interested in vision. He described the eye as part of an integrated, growing action system.

Eye muscles in children with developmental disabilities work very much the same way as the muscles in the rest of their bodies. So, if a child with spasticity moves his arms and legs slowly, with great effort, and without full range of motion, his eyes also will move more slowly. It will be hard to keep up with other children in the classroom at finding the right place in a book or on a chalkboard. If a child with athetosis has involuntary movements of her arms and legs, she probably will have trouble focusing her eyes while reading or following words while writing.

Most of these children don't have good alignment of body parts because of muscle pairs that aren't in balance. Eye muscles also have this problem, so one eye might drift out or in (crossed eyes). In order to see, children must be able to move their eyes easily, without effort, so that they can concentrate on identifying what they see. They also might need glasses in order to focus. A good eye exam will determine whether the child needs glasses. Some children's eyes might need surgery to line up the eyes correctly.

We can help our children give their eyes practice in working together and with the entire body during everyday activities. How can parents and other family members help? First, we must understand normal development and how babies learn to use their eyes. Here are a few examples:

- The infant looks toward the sound of Mom or Dad's voice (finding a target).
- During feeding, her eyes stay in one place (looking at the caregiver).
- His eyes are attracted to family members moving around the room (following the movements).
- When two different people talk to her, she looks first at one and then the other (shifting back and forth).

The baby spends 6 months practicing localization (finding a target), fixation (staying there long enough to determine what or who the target is), ocular pursuit (following the target when it moves), and gaze shifts (switching from one target to another).

All of these skills first happen in supine (on the back), where the head and body are totally supported. The eyes and head move together at first. Gradually the eyes learn to move separately from the head. As the baby lifts his head in prone (on the stomach) and develops head control, eye movements improve without the total environmental base of support. Eventually, the eyes become very skillful in other positions (sitting, standing, and walking). Moving the eyes separately from the head is very important for reading quickly and carefully.

Motor development affects vision and vice versa. An infant begins to focus on targets that are close when her own hand accidentally waves in front of her face. But seeing a toy that is out of reach makes a baby want to reach and grab it. So movement helps develop vision, and vision helps develop movement.

Children need more than near vision. They need to be aware of everything going on around them. Normally, this awareness begins when infants are startled and blink at something coming toward their faces quickly and unexpectedly. This is important for safety reasons, such as when we close the eyes to avoid being hurt. They gradually notice more and more, to their left and right sides and in front. Just as we need this visual skill to drive a car safely, children must notice and avoid obstacles when driving wheelchairs, especially powered ones. We also can offer children opportunities to get the kind of stimulation experiences they might have missed because of developmental delays and/or atypical movement patterns.

Neuro-Developmental Treatment (NDT) Principles

NDT principles can be very helpful in planning stimulation. When therapists and parents understand the reasons for doing certain activities, they can be creative in adapting them and thinking of new ones.

Here are some of those principles, along with simple ideas for improving how a child uses his or her eyes during everyday positioning, handling, and play. Most of these suggestions apply to babies and children who are very developmentally delayed, but you can adapt them for older children and those with milder delays.

- **NDT Principle:** Normal movement requires good body alignment and an active base of support so that muscles and joints can work most efficiently.

  Activity: Positioning and toy suggestions

  Method: If your child can't move easily by himself, change his position frequently so that he doesn't always turn his head and eyes only in one direction (toward the light from the same window or movement from someone coming in the door). Whether he is in bed, in a chair, or on the floor, alternate him from his left to his right side.

  Talk about where he is and the different things he can see from each place. Use wind chimes, prisms, scarves, fish tanks, birdcages or birdfeeders, mirrors, wind-up mobiles, and decorated paper plates (black and white, brightly colored).

  Use only one or two displays at a time to avoid overstimulation, and change them often. Show or help your child with hand clapping and finger plays. Let him explore puppets, tape, or yarn. Using both hands and eyes with the head in midline will improve his body symmetry.

- **NDT Principle:** Development or skill acquisition relies on the interaction of the body's many systems, its neural maturation, and interaction with the environment.

  Activity: Hide-and-seek and peek-a-boo games

  Method: Surprise your child by approaching her from different areas (the left and right sides, above and below, far and near). This will strengthen her defensive blink and help sharpen visual awareness of her surroundings.

- **NDT Principle:** Parents and other family members are important members of the team.

  Activity: Face-to-face interaction for eye contact and imitation

  Method: Encourage your child to take turns talking with you, not only with sounds, but also with facial expressions and hand movements (waving, clapping). Link the sound of your voice talking and singing with the movement of your mouth, eyes, and head. Wait patiently for him to respond before you continue each turn-taking moment.

- **NDT Principle:** Distal mobility depends on active or supported stability of the head and trunk.

  Activity: Following large and small moving targets (people, toys, food)

  Method: Give your child's head plenty of support in supine, supported sitting, or side lying, so that it is easier for her to control her eye movements. Put the target where the child can see it, then move it slowly enough so that she can keep on watching it. Use your voice or toys with sound to help her, but also try it without sound. Move a flashlight on the wall in a slightly darkened room. These activities will help the child's eyes move separately from her head.

- **NDT Principle:** Learning occurs during goal-directed activities that are motivated by pleasure.

  Activity: Manipulating toys for eye-hand coordination

  Method: Attach bells to elastic wrist and ankle bracelets on your baby so that he can combine looking and reaching with cause-and-effect touching. Suspend elastic across the crib or chair tray and attach manipulative toys to it. Look through your kitchen and dresser drawers for a variety of safe, interesting objects of different sizes, shapes, sounds, and textures (bracelets, key chains, measuring spoons, rubber gaskets, cloths, sponges). An older child can benefit from exploratory water play, sitting in the bathtub or standing at the sink, in a stander if necessary.

- **NDT Principle:** Key points of control (where you put your hands) help the baby move and have more normal sensations of movement. As the baby develops control, your hands give less assistance. Repetition helps the new movements become automatic and easy (new habits).

  Activity: Prone positioning

  Method: Carry your baby in prone suspension (stomach down), providing support wherever needed (stomach, chest, shoulders). Take tours of the house and neighborhood and talk about what you see. Play with her prone over your lap as she looks down at a mirror on the floor. Head control for downward gaze is necessary for eating, dressing, reading, and writing skills.

Precautions

Watch for signs of sensory overload or visual fatigue such as yawning, eye rubbing, eye rolling, blinking, irritability, or avoiding eye contact. Adapt activities by reducing how long you stimulate, how intense the stimulation is, or how many sensory channels are being stimulated simultaneously (sight, sound, touch, movement, and even taste and smell).

Summary

Parents can combine activities with touch and movement (rocking, patting, stroking, kissing), according to each child's tolerance and needs. Vision is one of the first ways babies learn about their world. When they link vision with the other senses, their developing brains take that information, sort it into categories, and store it to find later.

This important process leads to building knowledge, thinking, and making intelligent decisions. Children who can't move around to touch objects don't have the chance to link those experiences with matching visual information, so both their visual and motor development suffer. Parents, however, have many natural, enjoyable opportunities to stimulate visual-motor development in their babies and their older children during everyday positioning, handling, and play at home.

Adapted with permission from: Erhardt, R. P. (1991-1992, Winter). Improving visual control: Activities for parents and infants. *Team Talk, 1,* 12-15 (available from Team Talk, P.O. Box 83165, Milwaukee, WI 53223).

For more clarification of Neuro-Developmental Treatment (NDT) theory and how it influences therapy for children, see Article 1.2 by Judith Bierman, titled "Philosophy, Theory, and Principles: The What, Why, and How of NDT."

Buoyancy-Assisted Function Through Therapeutic Aquatics

Jane Styer-Acevedo, PT

"Hey, look at me, I'm swimming!" We hear this happy shout often in our swimming pools from children who have a difficult time moving on land, which is an environment where gravity is constantly pulling our bodies down. Resisting that pull is a challenge for all of us, but even more so for children with muscle weakness or stiffness. Unlike most children who move for the pleasure of movement itself, children with muscle problems learn that movement through space is a chore to be endured. So, how can water help us? How does it make it easier for us to move? Why do we enjoy it so much? We can find the answers to these questions by examining the actual physical properties of water, the effects of it on our movement, and how water play can be therapeutic.

Many therapists who work with children who have physical impairments use the Neuro-Developmental Treatment (NDT) philosophy. This hands-on approach includes current theories of motor learning and motor control that state that performance of a task is based on the interaction of the person, the environment, and the functional task requirements. Swimming and water play are popular functional activities that can be adapted to minimize impairments and build on strengths.

Safety

Water adjustment

It's important for children to have positive experiences very early in their contact with the pool. An easy way to decrease fear is to play with sponges and buckets of water on the pool deck. This allows the child to adjust to the area. You might initially choose to use a baby pool on the deck for water play.

Precautions

Children with stomas such as a *G tube* or *J tube* can go into the pool as long as the stoma is healthy and pink. If the site is oozing or open and raw, the child needs to wait until the stoma is healthy before entering the pool. I don't take children who have tracheotomies into the pool due to the very high risk of aspiration from splashing water.

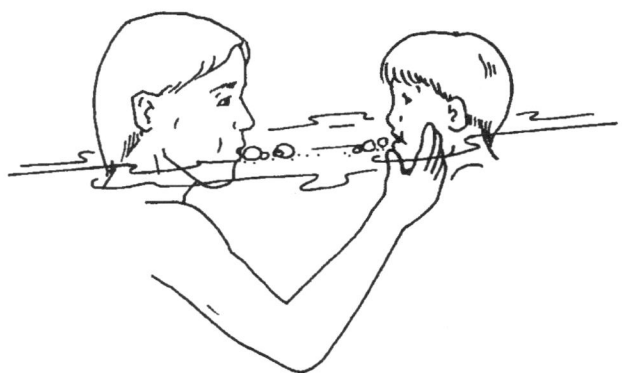

Figure 1. Support the lower jaw while demonstrating bubble blowing through the mouth. Slowly lower the child into the water until the mouth is covered.

Therapeutic warmth is 92° to 94° Fahrenheit. If your child gets cold in lower temperatures, leotards and tights or socks and a tight T-shirt might help insulate the body and hold in the warmth. While your child is in the pool, watch for any changes in breathing, skin color, and eyes, which reflect state changes such as:

- increased or decreased fear
- increased or decreased body temperature
- increased relaxation
- increased arousal
- improved breathing pattern followed by better floating and sometimes longer sentences and louder voices

Oral-motor control

Be cautious. Water can be a dangerous place for the child with imperfect breath control or limited oral-motor control, and your child shouldn't ingest large volumes of pool water. However, the pool is a great place to work on oral-motor control in the following ways:

- Support the lower jaw if the child can't get the lips closed, and demonstrate how to blow bubbles as you lower the child's lips (but not the nose!) into the water (Figure 1).
- Hold a straw and blow bubbles with it.
- Blow a Ping-Pong ball across the surface of the water.
- Sing or hum with the mouth under water.

Buoyancy-Assisted Function Through Therapeutic Aquatics

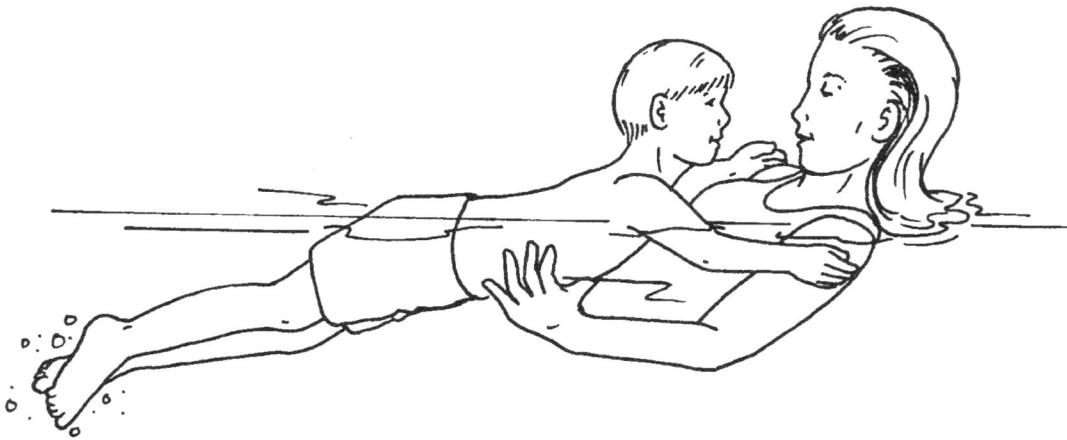

Figure 2. Placing your hands on the child's waist will help her to recover to vertical from a cheek-to-cheek position.

All these activities can improve lip closure, which is important for cleaning the spoon in feeding and saying the *b, p,* and *m* sounds.

Floating on the back: Recovery to vertical

The easiest way to help your child while she is on her back is the cheek-to-cheek position. Place her head on your shoulder so that your cheeks are touching. Your hands are now free to hold her waist or hips. This will greatly decrease fear. To sit up or stand, place your hand on her tummy and say, "chin tuck, knees to chest, feet to floor." Your hands can help her belly muscles work (Figure 2). When she brings her knees up, her hips will sink and her body will rotate to a vertical position. Your child eventually might learn to do this on her own. Floating should progress to where her head no longer is on your shoulder but rather in front of you.

Floating on the tummy: Recovery to vertical

You can practice this type of floating before putting your child's face in the water if you provide support. Initially, ask the child to place his hands on your shoulders when facing you (Figure 3). Your hands can support his tummy. Use similar words, "knees to chest, head up, feet to floor," to rotate him to vertical. Your hands again will help the tummy muscles. Your child can become progressively more independent with this float by:

- holding on to the side of the pool
- supporting himself on a kickboard with his hands
- floating with his face in the water and blowing bubbles before recovering to vertical

Physical Properties of Water

Buoyancy

Buoyancy is the force in the water that is constantly pushing us up toward the surface of the water, opposite to the force of gravity. If the two forces are exactly equal and opposite, we will float with no rotation—that is, flat on the surface of the water (Figure 4a). Everyone can float. The size and shape of our bodies determine where (floating on or under the surface) and how (rotating side to side or top to bottom, Figure 4b).

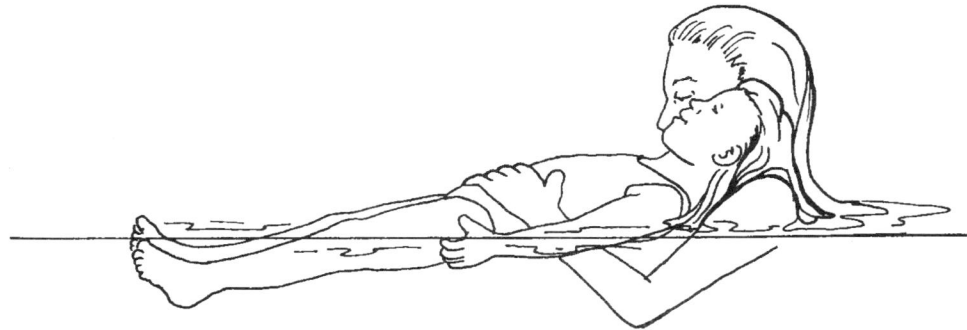

Figure 3. Have the child push on your shoulders or chest while facing you in order to practice kicking while on his tummy. Your hands can help his belly work to get his knees under him.

Buoyancy-Assisted Function Through Therapeutic Aquatics

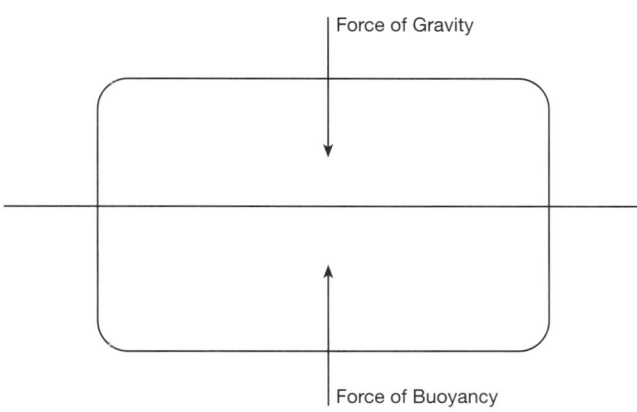

Figure 4a. When the effect of the force of gravity equals the effect of the force of buoyancy, the body will float flat on the surface of the water.

Because buoyancy is a welcomed assist that decreases gravity's downward pull on our bodies, we love to play and swim in the water. This often is the vehicle needed to equalize the child with nondisabled peers. Suddenly the child can do the same or similar things as friends and siblings, with little extra effort. What a booster for morale and self-esteem! Bear in mind that the force of buoyancy always is pushing toward the surface of the water. If a child tries to retrieve a submerged toy, he will be working *against* the force of buoyancy. For example, flutter kicking while on the back, as in a back crawl, makes the muscles of the buttocks work against buoyancy. This is great for the person who has trouble standing up straight due to weakness of this muscle group.

You can select activities that provide gradually more resistive exercise in the water. These activities can take the form of exercises, activities, games, swimming, and even walking. Wearing an air-filled flotation device while moving and exercising in the water will change the amount of work the child must do. A water wing around the wrist or ankle helps bring the arm or leg to the surface. Placing that same arm or leg back under the water requires the child to work against the force of buoyancy. When you change the amount of air in the flotation device, you can provide the child with multiple levels of progressive resistive exercises.

We all have an internal flotation device as well—our lungs. Altering the amount of air we hold in our lungs will change the way we float and move in the water.

Water rresistance

Water resistance is called hydrostatic pressure. As pressure gives resistance to movement in water, it also assists with movement. Imagine yourself walking through water up to your chest. Suddenly you stub your toe on an object. You begin to fall, but it takes a relatively long time for your face to hit the water, compared with falling on the sidewalk. This resistance is exceedingly helpful to the child with poor balance who has difficulty walking independently on land. Supported by the water, the child has more time to learn what the correct balance response should be when balance is challenged. Walking in increasingly shallow water as balance improves will lead toward improved function on land. A simple progression is for your child to:

- step on your feet under the water and keep them down as you "dance" together
- walk in the water while holding your hands
- cruise along the side of the pool
- walk in the water holding a foam noodle or kickboard in front for support (vary the water depth from shoulder level to hip level)
- walk independently in increasingly shallow water

Resistance always increases as the speed of movement increases. This is similar to doing resistive exercises on land but is much more fun! Try challenging the child in a playful manner to do the activity faster—to run instead of

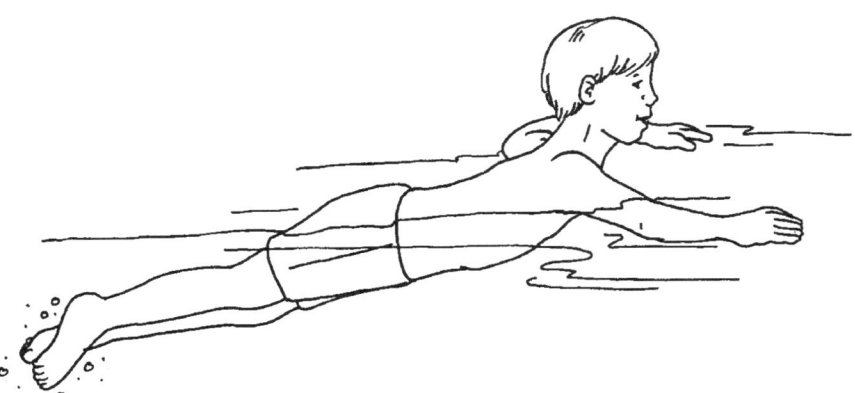

Figure 4b. When the effect of the force of gravity does not equal the effect of the force of buoyancy, the body will rotate and find its equilibrium.

walk, swim faster, take giant steps instead of baby steps, catch a ball before it hits the water, or retrieve a weighted ring before it sinks to the pool floor.

Turbulence

Another way to increase the work of movement in water is to increase the turbulence through which one is moving. Splash and churn the water around the child as she plays a game of catch or walks to retrieve a floating object. This will challenge her balance and strengthen her muscles in a fun way. Encourage the child to splash back at you. See who can splash the most! This added resistance to the arm muscles will strengthen them. This splashing game also is an effective way to decrease tactile sensitivity (the fear or dislike of being touched).

Moving your child quickly through the water in a horizontal or vertical position increases the turbulence and therefore how the child perceives and adjusts to touch. Add fun sounds such as "swoosh," "swish," or motorboat sounds to increase the pleasure. If your child is water safe with good oral-motor control, gently throw him into the air and splash him back into the water, or toss him to someone standing 2 or 3 feet away from you. Or, he can jump independently, pushing off from your legs into someone else's arms. These actions wake up the body by increasing tactile input as well as joint receptor input (proprioception).

Swimming Strokes

It is important to choose the swim stroke that is the most therapeutic for the child (not necessarily the easiest one). Working on that stroke routinely will help the child develop a sense of accomplishment as it becomes easier and function on land improves. It could be a stroke that lengthens short muscles or strengthens those that are weak. It could decrease stiffness because it incorporates rotation of the trunk or limbs. The stroke might lengthen the short side of the trunk and limbs of a child with hemiplegia. The child will need help and encouragement because the appropriate stroke undoubtedly will be difficult at first.

It's important to remember that the easiest stroke for the child actually might increase a deformity already present or threatening to appear. A good example would be a child who has a problem with rounded shoulders and shortened chest muscles. A front crawl might be easiest, but an elementary back stroke or back crawl would lengthen the chest muscles with every stroke taken. Hurray!

Integration of Land and Water Activities

Water can be both fun and therapeutic. When used effectively, it can improve function on land in some of the following ways:

- strengthening tummy muscles to improve breathing, making talking easier, sentences longer, and voices louder
- strengthening tummy muscles and working on balance in progressively shallower water, followed by practice on land to make walking more efficient on land
- doing a flutter kick while holding onto the wall or a kickboard to strengthen shoulder muscles and improve hand grasp
- learning to blow bubbles for improved lip closure to clean a spoon while eating and even to blow kisses

Group Participation

Peer group activities usually are very motivating to children, especially when playing in the water allows them to move more freely and easily than on land. Successful games and activities include Ring Around the Rosie, Simon Says, tag, beach volleyball, water basketball, and the simple catching and throwing of balls of all sizes. Also competition between groups and individuals can be healthy and motivating. It can be as simple as seeing who can get to the wall the fastest by any means possible, or it can be organized competition as structured as the Special Olympics. The child must be well matched to the group and activity to ensure success.

Swimming is *fun*! It is an equalizer for the child adversely effected by gravity. It is a means of expression and independence for the child who has significant motor and sensory impairments. It can help bring a family together and include a child who generally has difficulty participating in group or family activities. It is a therapeutic, regular, everyday activity that includes, rather than excludes, the child. Use it and enjoy!

For more clarification of Neuro-Developmental Treatment (NDT) theory and how it influences therapy for children, see Article 1.2 by Judith Bierman, titled "Philosophy, Theory, and Principles: The What, Why, and How of NDT."

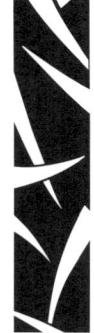

Hippotherapy: Treatment With the Help of the Horse

Linda Kliebhan, PT

Children with movement disorders such as cerebral palsy who receive therapy services from early in life or for long periods of time often reach a point where they need something new and different, something exciting that helps them stay motivated to work hard. Therapeutic horseback riding is a wonderful way to keep kids moving toward their therapy-program goals, and it benefits the whole child—body, mind, and spirit.

The physical benefits of therapeutic riding include positive effects on muscles, joints, balance, endurance, and respiration (control of breathing). Many guiding principles of therapeutic riding are similar to the principles of Neuro-Developmental Treatment (NDT), which your child already might be receiving, so the two complement each other and can be combined very easily.

Because different types of horseback riding can be therapeutic, parents need to distinguish among them in order to choose the right program for their child.

Some types of therapeutic riding are available as individual physical, occupational, or speech-therapy sessions. Other types take place individually or in groups and may be led by a trained riding instructor who is not a therapist. Programs that provide individual physical therapy, occupational therapy, or speech therapy usually aren't aimed at teaching children how to ride, so it's important to consider what your child is ready for, and match his or her needs to the program you choose.

Hippotherapy is the term used for a method of treatment that was developed in Germany more than 30 years ago. The term, which has been used throughout Europe and the United States, means "treatment with the help of the horse." The oldest form of hippotherapy (sometimes called classic hippotherapy) uses the horse as the primary therapy tool, as if the horse were a piece of therapy equipment such as a therapy ball or a bolster.

Horses are chosen for hippotherapy based on gentleness, tolerance, and the quality of their movements. The child reacts to the movement of the horse with improved posture and movement responses. As the horse walks, the horse's body moves in up and down, forward and back, side to side, and in rotational directions. These movements occur over and over and transfer to the child. The movements are very similar to some of the movements a person uses during normal walking.

The child might sit on the horse facing forward or backward or lie on the back or the stomach. A bareback pad and various types of surcingles (handles) are the only equipment used, so that the child feels the movement of the horse and the warmth of the horse's body. A specially trained therapist (physical or occupational therapist or speech-language pathologist) directs the person leading the horse to adjust the horse's speed and movement and to change those directions constantly, based on the child's responses.

Another type of therapeutic riding combines classic hippotherapy with specific principles of physical, occupational, or speech therapy, or psychology. The therapist chooses horses for their specific characteristics that will facilitate the goals of each child and selects activities on the horse to focus on specific therapy goals. The session might include equipment such as a saddle or stirrups attached to the surcingle. For example, the therapist might ask a child to move from sit to stand on the horse repetitively, in order to strengthen leg muscles, stretch tight heel cords, and/or improve balance in order to improve the child's ability to walk. The therapist might ask the child to maintain a hands-and-knees position on the horse as it moves in order to increase sensory input, weight bearing, and control of postural muscles in the shoulders, trunk, and hips. The functional goal might be crawling on all fours or supporting weight on the arms for other tasks such as pushing a walker.

Some hippotherapy programs include additional therapy time off the horse. Before mounting the horse, the child might do stretching exercises as a warm-up. After dismounting, those same types of exercises help transfer activities on the horse into daily living activities. For example, a child might help brush the horse to increase range of reach with the arms as well as standing balance. Another example would be reaching for objects in sitting after getting off the horse, using the improved trunk control gained from sitting on the horse.

Developmental Riding Therapy is another form of therapeutic riding, usually done individually. It differs from hippotherapy in that it includes aspects of horsemanship, including learning to ride. This type of program might be appropriate for children who have met the goals of their hippotherapy programs but might not be ready for therapeutic group riding, or for those whose physical impairments do not require hippotherapy.

Last but not least, many recreational therapeutic riding programs emphasize basic riding skills and the enjoyment of riding. These programs also have therapeutic benefits. They use trained riding instructors, with therapists acting as consultants in some cases.

All therapeutic riding programs require a team of trained personnel that includes specially trained therapists, horse experts, and lots of volunteers to ensure safety. Reputable programs require a physician's referral even if the program is not billed as therapy. Volunteers may act as side-walkers for safety or they may be involved in tacking the horses (getting the horse ready, putting on pads or saddles). Volunteers must be trained, but they don't necessarily need extensive experience with horses or riding. Volunteering offers a terrific way for parents, siblings, or other family members and friends to be involved in the child's program.

You will need to consider several factors if you are thinking about enrolling your child in a therapeutic riding program:

- Most children are not able to participate until they are 4 or 5 years of age.
- Therapy goals should be consistent with movements that can be accomplished on the horse.
- Always consult a physician to make sure there are no medical reasons precluding participation.

NDT Principles

Most forms of therapeutic riding are consistent with the basic theory and many of the principles of NDT.

- **NDT Principle:** Body alignment is a critical component of functional tasks.

    Therapeutic Riding: The size of the horse, the quality of the horse's movement, and the activities used on the horse naturally facilitate the alignment of the child's spine and hips similar to that required for sitting, standing, and walking.

- **NDT Principle:** Postural control is an integral part of movement and is learned through experience.

    Therapeutic Riding: The movement of the horse automatically requires the child to activate postural muscles. The specific direction and speed of movement, as well as the positions used, can help the child learn postural responses that prepare for, accompany, or react to movement, all of which are aspects of integrated postural control that are necessary for functional skills.

- **NDT Principle:** The ability to activate postural muscles against the supporting surface is essential for efficient functional motor control.

    Therapeutic Riding: The majority of activities and postures assumed on the horse require the child to activate against the base of support (the horse) and to sustain that activity for periods of time. The child can do this both when the horse is standing still (nonmovable surface) and when the horse is moving (movable surface).

Summary

Many different types of therapeutic horseback riding are available for children with movement disorders, including classic hippotherapy, hippotherapy, and developmental riding. Therapists can use these activities as alternatives to, or in combination with, the traditional model of physical, occupational, or speech therapy. The horse becomes a tool to achieve similar goals, and the techniques chosen depend on the type of approach used and the individual needs of the child.

Therapeutic riding affects many different systems and considers the whole child. In addition to the physical benefits it provides improved motivation, the development of self-esteem, and independence.

For more clarification of Neuro-Developmental Treatment (NDT) theory and how it influences therapy for children, see Article 1.2 by Judith Bierman, titled "Philosophy, Theory, and Principles: The What, Why, and How of NDT."

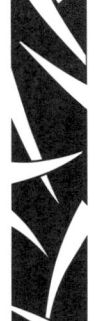

Getting Pumped Up for Therapy During the Teen Years: Working Through the Stress of Adolescence

Madonna Nash, OTR

"Therapy is boring. I'm ready to quit. When can I graduate? I've been in therapy since I was born!"

These are just a few comments and concerns from adolescents who have functional limitations and impairments that occur as a result of cerebral palsy.

Adolescence is the transition between childhood and adulthood, generally spanning from 11 to 19 years of age. As the child reaches adolescence, body image, self-concept, and a sense of self become more important than at any other age. Major physical, intellectual, and psychosocial changes occur that are quite different from early childhood. It is a time of rapid growth, body consciousness, and appearance of sexual maturity. Teenagers are trying to come to some acceptance of body type as well as physical assets and deficits. In order to develop an integrated body image of him- or herself as a unique person, the adolescent needs to resolve issues of identity, self-esteem, and emotional independence from parents, and determine the direction of future plans. Other critical social-emotional behaviors include peer interaction, the development of significant social relationships, feedback from peers, involvement in sports or dance to enhance physical skill and coordination, and participation in scholastic and extracurricular activities (organized clubs, scouts).

In addition to these changes that occur in teens without disabilities, the developing adolescent with cerebral palsy also might have to deal with increased joint and muscle pain and stress, decline in mobility due to bone and muscle mass, and increased fatigue.

It is critical that exercise be increased rather than eliminated at this stage of development because it is so easy for adolescents to become sedentary. We cannot allow exercise to be an option; instead, it must become a critical part of the challenged teen's daily life skills. We must optimize their involvement and performance in movement activities to prevent physical impairments from developing into handicapping conditions.

One of the most significant impairments that concerns therapists is muscle weakness, especially in cerebral palsy. When prolonged, this weakness leads to inefficient movement and a growing number of functional limitations that add to the list of secondary impairments (compensations) and deformity. By the time they reach the teen years, many adolescents have had some type of surgical intervention, which also increases the possibility of muscle weakness. As a consequence, additional secondary impairments sometimes include isolation from social opportunities, low self-expectations, increased difficulty managing daily life tasks, and the resulting depression if social-emotional needs are not met.

How do parents help therapists understand and respect the child's wishes to decrease or change the form of their therapy when those therapists understandably are concerned about the rapid growth changes associated with adolescence and the impairments associated with cerebral palsy?

Many families' lifestyles don't include regular exercise programs. Although we realize that this is their choice, from a therapist's point of view, children with disabilities really don't have a choice. They have predetermined motor impairments with predictable compensations that place them at a disadvantage for motor activities that their nonchallenged peers can partake in automatically. Exercise for these children is critical, and they have so much to gain.

Parents often ask, "What do they have to gain? What are they going to get out of this? Why is this important?"

Statistically, people who exercise have an increased life expectancy and can decrease the potential for many disease processes—heart disease, cancer, obesity, and high blood pressure. The immune system is less susceptible to illness when we exercise, which means fewer trips to the doctor. The digestive system, bowel, and bladder function better with regular exercise.

A routine exercise program can be an outlet for aggression and frustration, which leads to fewer mood swings. In recent years, there has been a surge in the interest in pediatric exercise medicine. Studies done with adolescents who have neuromotor problems indicate that physical activity programs improve motor skills in cerebral palsy. Skeletal muscle adapts to changes in habitual exercise by alterations in structure and function. Spasticity is associated with structural changes in the muscle that result in metabolic inefficiency, fatigue, and altered muscle mechanical properties. Adolescents with physical impairments should be afforded similar opportunities in movement activities as their nonchallenged peers. However, due to the constraints of their movement disorders, many of these activities are difficult or require a greater period of time to learn.

A majority of parents don't have time to do all this. However, therapists and parents have an important responsibility to provide children with opportunities so that they can be the best they can be. Therapists trained in Neuro-Developmental Treatment (NDT) are sensitive to the sensory and motor impairments and the functional and societal limitations that occur in the developing adolescent with neuromotor problems. We can implement programs that decrease the effect of muscle weakness, build endurance, and promote self-esteem and confidence. A knowledge of fitness for adolescents with cerebral palsy can provide information regarding functional limitations and determine the effects and benefits of therapeutic intervention. Poor physical fitness compromises daily life function and social integration. Affected components include muscle strength (the maximal force that can be generated at a given joint angle), peak muscle power (the highest mechanical work performed per unit of time), muscle endurance (the ability to sustain work or power at a high intensity), and maximal aerobic power. Many therapists have implemented programs in their hospital settings and private practices to optimize adolescents' exercise programs. These provide meaningful, context-specific activities that motivate and engage the developing adolescent and assist in realization of functional goals. Participating in an organized exercise program that is adapted for the adolescent with special needs can assist in alignment, stability, mobility, strength, and endurance during growth and maturation. It can prevent health-risk factors such as obesity and other degenerative diseases. Proper exercise and fitness is the single most factor in preventing injuries.

Parents might ask, "If my child can't bike or use Roller Blades®, how can I help the child increase aerobic capacity when we're not in therapy?"

Some of the programs that commonly have been implemented as an adjunct to therapy programs are martial arts, dance/dance therapy, low-impact aerobics (cycling, treadmill, Stairmaster®), and weight training. Offering these options to your child can allow him or her to choose an activity that stimulates interest. Motivation and enthusiasm are the keys to maintaining an exercise program on a regular basis.

NDT Principles

The following current NDT principles serve as a rationale for implementation of programs that support physical fitness of the adolescent.

- **NDT Principle:** Postural control and movement components are learned through practice and experience.

  Activity: Dance therapy

  Method: Dance therapy is defined as the psychotherapeutic use of movement, based on the assumption that mind and body are in constant reciprocal interaction. Movement therapy bridges the gap between the body and the mind. We know that body language is more powerful than verbal communication. This has great impact on adolescents who have difficulty with nonverbal communication. Activities include posture, movement, music, mime, gesture, story, and drama.

- **NDT Principle:** Motor development requires changes that seek new and more adaptive movement configurations that are context-specific (based upon the dynamical systems approach). Motor patterns vary with age across the life span. Structure and function constantly shape each other; the environment and task affect this function.

  Activity: Dance

  Method: Ballet, jazz, modern, tap, African, and the Irish step dance are some of the popular forms that the adolescent can enjoy. These various styles of dance can emphasize a wide variety of movement components and facilitate a variety of postural-control issues. Performance in a recital can enhance confidence, self-worth, and self-esteem.

- **NDT Principle:** Human beings are motivated by functional task goals. The key to success of intervention is motivation to be actively involved. In addition, participation in community recreational activities increases physical capabilities (strength, coordination, and endurance), self-esteem, and body image.

  Activity: Martial arts/karate

  Method: Each of the martial arts has a spiritual component that teaches students self-esteem, self-respect, and body awareness. Being physically and mentally fit builds self-confidence. Karate consists primarily of striking, blocking, and kicking tech-niques that use the upper and lower extremities. It is a challenging way to develop strength, flexibility, and self-defense.

- **NDT Principle:** Normal postural control is the organized product of engagement in functional, oriented tasks. A hallmark of efficient motor function is that the individual can combine an infinite number of movements into desired functional activities in a wide variety of environmental conditions.

  Activity: Tai Chi

  Method: Tai Chi is a series of slow-moving exercises performed smoothly and accurately with relaxed muscles and the mind absorbed in the movement. It emphasizes a stress-free mind and a flexible body. In addition, it stimulates the internal organs, exercises the body, calms the nervous system, and mobilizes the joints.

- **NDT Principle:** The basis of treatment is the utilization of facilitation techniques to improve lengthening of the muscles (flexibility), eccentric/concentric control of the muscles (lengthening and shortening) during functional tasks, and activation of synergies (groups of muscles that work together for functional purposes). These improvements promote movement strategies and the strengthening of weak muscles to enhance motor control.

  Activity: Using exercise equipment

  Method: Aerobic endurance and muscular strength are the easiest fitness components to improve. Treadmills, stair steppers, stationary bikes, and weight training programs are motivating for the adolescent and enhance endurance, physical activity, and mechanical efficiency, which usually are diminished in the adolescent who deals with poor muscle tone, postural regulation, and involuntary movements.

Summary

Adolescents with neuromotor disorders need opportunities to maximize aerobic power and enhance their physical activity level. Families and therapists should collaborate to establish physical fitness programs that support the adolescent's daily life function, self-esteem, and social integration. Maintaining flexibility, strength, alignment, and active movement through activity are important factors in preventing cardiovascular disease and reducing the risk of high blood pressure and obesity. Exercise improves self-confidence and self-image as well as balance and coordination, which allow greater ease and efficiency in the performance of motor tasks. Managing health and well-being is the key to becoming self-sufficient, maintaining independence, and enjoying full participation in society.

For more clarification of Neuro-Developmental Treatment (NDT) theory and how it influences therapy for children, see Article 1.2 by Judith Bierman, titled "Philosophy, Theory, and Principles: The What, Why, and How of NDT."

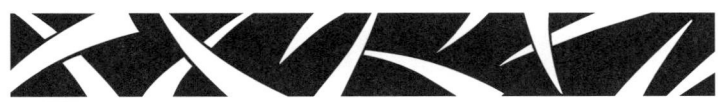

Section 7

Communication and School Activities

To Speak Is the Greatest Gift: Facilitating Oral-Motor Coordination for Speech Production

Merry M. Meek, M.S., CCC-Sp

Speech is a very complex motor activity that allows us one means of expressing ourselves. We also express ourselves with our facial, arm, and hand gestures as well as whole-body movement. The prerequisite for expression is understanding what language is—which means having something to say and being motivated to use everything we have to get our message across.

In order to use speech, we have to coordinate our respiration pattern (particularly exhalation) with phonation (making a sound). Then we must articulate sounds with the movements of the jaw, cheeks, lips, and tongue. To say words requires greater coordination of these movements. All of these movements require oral-motor and respiratory control. Often, the child cannot make a sound easily due to short, shallow breathing and poor coordination of the movements in the vocal folds and mouth. This creates more problems in words that require a combination of several sounds, such as "bye bye" or "Hi, mama."

Vocalization can be more difficult for children who have neurological problems with body alignment and movement control in the body. It is the stability and control within the trunk and shoulder girdle that assist good breathing and phonation. Stability and control of the head and neck allow the jaw to use fine movements to coordinate with cheeks, lips, and tongue musculature.

We can help children learn to talk by cueing the movements of the mouth to make different sounds and by positioning them to give their bodies alignment symmetry and stability, and facilitate better coordination of breathing with phonation.

Within the first few months of life, normal babies begin to practice cooing sounds that are vowel-like in nature (*ah, oo,* and *ae,* as they cry). From 4 months of age, they play with blowing air (exhalation), combined with consonants (*mm, babe,* and lip/tongue "raspberries"). As they develop more jaw grading with chewing at about 6 months and older, we start to hear more tongue movement sounds (*da, ta-ta, la-la, na-na*) or even the beginnings of *no-no*. Generally between 9 and 12 months, we hear these same sounds bridging to words. Thanks to their language development, we hear children say "mama," "dada," and "baba" (which can represent "bottle," "baby," "ball," or "bye-bye," depending on the situation).

Other important steps toward learning to talk are imitating sounds and taking turns vocalizing, which are heard usually in the 9- to 12-month period and quite dramatically by 18 months, when they copy words they shouldn't hear.

We can help children coordinate these activities as we:

- hold them and talk to them in a way that they can watch our facial movements
- develop their feeding skills, which use similar motor movement patterns
- position them to facilitate language development, so that they can see, touch, and hear the names of animals, toys, foods, and the action or verbs (doggie eat, throw ball)
- give touch/kinesthetic cues around the mouth to facilitate jaw, cheek, lip, and tongue movement for specific sounds

Neuro-Developmental Treatment (NDT) Principles

The following guidelines describe NDT principles and ideas to help the child make sounds and later combine them into words.

- **NDT Principle:** Normal movement requires good body alignment and a stable head position so the mouth can coordinate precise movements for vocalizing.

    Activity: Positioning and touch suggestions for mouth rounding (*oo, oa, w, u*)

    Method: The child needs a stable position for the head, neck, and shoulder girdle in order to watch your face as you help the child make the sounds by facilitating facial movement. Gradually stroke the child's cheeks with your hands so that the mouth appears more round. Say "oo, moo, toot, choo-choo, shoo, hoo-hoo, woof-woof" to encourage imitation.

- **NDT Principle:** Speech requires grading mouth opening and closure for consonants.

    Activity: Positioning and touch suggestions for sounds requiring mouth closure (*p, b, m, f, v*)

    Method: It is extremely important that your child's head/neck not pull back as you facilitate mouth closure, and that the neck not be in hyperextension. Placing one of your hands on the chest will encourage the chin-down position as the index and middle finger of your other hand gently move the chin up to the lower lip. With the child's mouth in this closed position, make *m, b,* and *p* sounds, or say "Big Bird, Barney, baby, bop, mama, bye" for your child to imitate. Use the index and middle fingers gently to move the lower lip slightly under the upper teeth as you say *f* and *v* and combine for simple words: "four, five, fun," or "fee, fie, foe, fum." Gradually open the mouth a little with the index and middle fingers as you say "ah ha, no no, hi, hey, eyum yum."

- **NDT Principle:** Proximal control allows for specific movements for distal mobility.

  Activity: Positioning and tongue-tip activity for *(d, t, n, l)* sounds

  Method: Maintain the child's head in a stable position with the head slightly more forward or looking down. This allows the tongue to come forward and be closer to the roof of the mouth where many tongue-tip sounds occur. Use your index finger to touch the middle of the child's upper lip slowly and firmly as you say "da, dada" or "daddy, dog, duck, down." Use your index finger to touch the middle of the upper lip lightly and quickly as you say "ta, tick tock, tee, toy, talk." Use your index finger on the middle of the upper lip with another finger gently touching the top of the nose as you say "na, no no, now, name, nae nae." Use your index finger stroking forward under the chin/tongue as you say "lala, lulu, lili," silly sounds like "bla, bla, la lee lee," and the words "love, like, light." Use your index finger circulating under the chin/tongue as you say "thth" or car motor sounds such as "errie, grr."

- **NDT Principle:** Proximal control allows for specific movements distally.

  Activity: Position and touch suggestions for guttural sounds *(k, g, ng)*

  Method: Place the child in a slightly reclined position so that the tongue falls back a little toward the throat. Gently use your thumb and index finger to push up under the chin against the base of the tongue as you say "ka ka, ga ga, cough, grr, cookie, cake, car, go, goat, gum, give."

Communication with one another for human contact and interaction is extremely important in the bonding and nurturing of children. Facilitating this communication process is very rewarding for the child and family.

For more clarification of Neuro-Developmental Treatment (NDT) theory and how it influences therapy for children, see Article 1.2 by Judith Bierman, titled "Philosophy, Theory, and Principles: The What, Why, and How of NDT."

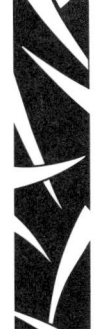

Reading: Opening Communication Interactions 7.2

Deborah Minteer, M.S., CCC-SLP

It might be difficult for you as a parent to know how to begin communication interactions with your child who has developmental disabilities and delays. You might be busy with daily care and might not know how to interact with this child whose communication skills are slow to develop.

Communication usually begins with parent-to-child eye contact and continues as parent and child interact with simple verbal interactions and continued eye contact. It is important that infants attend to facial expressions and hear spoken language. They learn to listen to the rate, rhythm, volume, and inflection of the human voice. Talking to young infants and describing to them the actions or events that occur during the day is like telling them the story of their lives. It's easy to do this during daily care. By talking to your child and giving him or her your undivided attention, you are beginning the communication loop of listening and responding and learning each other's communication signals. Children who have many opportunities to look at simple objects or pictures as you talk about them are developing important early attending skills that lead to the enjoyment of being read to and later reading for pleasure themselves.

Nursery rhymes, picture-only books, and very short stories help infants and young toddlers learn some of the basics of reading, such as holding a book and turning the pages. You probably already realize that children this age typically ask parents to read the same books over and over. Children enjoy stories that are short and have a simple rhyme or rhythm. Repetition is an important part of learning. You can further this learning by asking the child to point to or label with a single word the common objects and pictures within the story.

From about 3 to 5 years of age, children are very aware of the printed word and are excited about learning to read. They sometimes pretend to read books. You can increase your child's interest, skill, and enjoyment by trying these simple suggestions:

- Allow your child to read you a story or to join you while you read.
- Pause and let the child fill in the blanks. For example, "He huffed, and he puffed, and he blew the ____ down."
- Ask open-ended questions that encourage problem solving, such as, "What do you think will happen next?"
- Point to or move your finger under each word as you read. This helps preschoolers connect printed words to spoken words.
- Teach the letters of the alphabet and sing the ABC song. At this age children still enjoy books with rhymes and repetition.
- Add stories with simple plots.
- For children who have limited verbal skills, remember to allow time for a response. Accept the response and expand on it.
- If your child is unable to point or has limited pointing abilities, move the child's hand to the picture you describe and label it.
- If your child is limited in speech, accept what your child produces vocally and encourage even more use of the voice to allow more active participation in the reading activity.

Beginning readers (5 to 8 years old) like to see progress in their abilities. They learn best through repetition. Rereading short sentences or simple books helps children recognize words and later read more smoothly. Let your child share reading aloud. Take turns reading short sentences or you start reading a sentence and then wait for him to say a word that you know is familiar. If he tires or becomes discouraged, take over and continue reading to him.

Children who are 8 to 10 years old will combine strategies, using meaning and context to understand and sound out words they don't know. Their reading aloud still might sound choppy, but now they are interested in reading silently as well as doing more writing. If your child has a writing difficulty, help him write simple words and sentences. It's still a good time to choose books for your child that might seem too easy, but these actually will build the child's confidence. Encourage your child to catch her own reading errors while you listen to her read aloud. Don't stop reading aloud. Suggest that your child read to younger children, siblings, or friends, whenever possible. Remember to ask questions about what the child has read, which develops reading comprehension and understanding and keeps the focus on the content rather than just reading meaningless words.

Independent readers have mastered basic reading skills and have learned to teach themselves new things by reading. They now interpret what they read or read between the lines. You can encourage your child's reading by providing a steady flow of interesting books.

The child with neuromotor problems might find reading to be slow and difficult. Alternative activities and suggestions that can foster reading enjoyment include:

- Ask a peer, older child, or grandparent to read to the child. Encourage them to ask simple questions and wait for a response.
- Use books that are on tape, and purchase a tape recorder that is adaptable to switch use so that the child can access the story without help.
- Try adaptations such as Intellikeys® or key guards on computers. These adaptations help children become successful at reading stories on computer software.
- Both younger and older children enjoy having stories read to them in bed.
- Make reading a fun and interesting activity for your child and your. Ham it up! Use funny voices for character changes. Give the characters your child's name.
- Notice what interests your child, and have plenty of books, magazines, or comics from which to choose. Respect those choices.
- Go often to the library and find out about story hours for children. Begin to build your own library.
- Tell your child stories you remember from your childhood.
- If your child seems to be losing interest in a story, skip the parts that are too detailed.
- Describe interesting daily events to your child, and encourage him or her to do the same.
- Ask questions. Wait for responses.
- Take turns reading aloud.
- Always provide a sense of completion. If you aren't able to finish the story, find an appropriate stopping point.

Neuro-Developmental Treatment (NDT) Principles

Principles of the NDT approach can be useful as a guide for parents with children who have developmental delays and neuromotor problems.

- **NDT Principle:** Appropriate positioning for the best possible alignment of the body is important, especially for eye, head, and arm function during reading.

    Activity: By positioning the child on your lap, you can assist with pointing. Don't be surprised if the very young child isn't interested in sitting still and listening for long periods of time. Encourage the preschool child to remain for longer attending periods and task completion. You can sit across from or next to the child who is older and in a wheelchair. This still allows for close contact during reading, and you can continue to assist with pointing. Use other seating systems to add variety.

- **NDT Principle:** The team approach includes the parents as part of the child's learning team.

    Activity: Being read to is an activity most children enjoy. It offers a time to stimulate language learning while providing opportunities for a child to express already-gained knowledge verbally.

- **NDT Principle:** Active participation from the child is a basic principle of the NDT approach.

    Activity: Reading can be an interactive activity that is fun for the child and the parent.

Books are an important part of learning. Reading to a child offers a wonderful opportunity for you and your child to sit together, talk to each other, and learn!

For more clarification of Neuro-Developmental Treatment (NDT) theory and how it influences therapy for children, see Article 1.2 by Judith Bierman, titled "Philosophy, Theory, and Principles: The What, Why, and How of NDT."

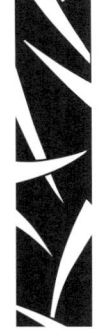

Layering: An Art of Therapy

Judy Michels Jelm, M.S., CCC-SLP

Parents often wonder how and why therapists use specific treatment techniques for their child.

During a treatment session, your physical therapist, occupational therapist, or speech-language pathologist chooses specific treatment techniques in response to your child's individual functional needs. Although your therapist organizes a specific treatment plan for your child prior to each session, that plan can change significantly during a session, depending on your child's response to a certain technique. A therapist also incorporates different techniques when a new discovery about your child becomes evident during a session.

Layering is an important concept that recognizes that treatment is a discovery process. During an archeological expedition, the archeologists use very specific tools such as shovels, picks, and brushes to uncover and discover the different layers of the earth. Every layer provides incredibly important information to the scientist. Similarly, the tools of discovery for the therapist are treatment techniques.

As your therapist interacts with you and your child, each of you will learn new information as your child begins to acquire new skills. As therapists make new discoveries, they modify the treatment strategies and techniques. It is a problem-solving process. If therapy strategies don't change as new information emerges, therapy can't be successful. A therapist who uses the Neuro-Developmental Treatment (NDT) approach recognizes that as your child changes, treatment techniques also must change to meet the special needs of your child.

For example, as a speech-language therapist, I treated a child who was diagnosed initially as verbally dyspraxic. This 3-year-old couldn't say very many sounds. He followed many age-appropriate directions but could not imitate any lip or tongue movements. Most speech therapists would expect that, at his age, he would easily be able to imitate a variety of lip and tongue movements.

I began to design specific treatment techniques for him based upon his initial diagnosis and aimed to meet his most predominant functional need—to be understood by others. With treatment, this child initially became aware of how to imitate lip movements during play activities and later learned how to imitate sounds that required the same movements of the lips. For example, he learned how to imitate lip rounding. He also learned how to vocalize the sound "o" and later learned how to use the "o" sound to say "o-pen." This child's ability to be understood improved consistently week after week.

As time progressed, I discovered a different problem area that hadn't been apparent previously. As this child was learning to imitate tongue movements, his tongue appeared to be moving differently from before. His tongue appeared to be moving much slower to the left than to the right side of his mouth. His mom also commented that he was becoming a very sloppy eater. The movements of his tongue now were preventing him from making sounds that demanded precise, quick tongue movements. In speech therapy terms, an underlying layer of mild dysarthria was now evident. The mild dysarthria probably had been there all the time, but it had been masked by the significant problem area of verbal dyspraxia. As the original problem area began to improve, the underlying problem became more predominant. With the discovery of this new layer, we incorporated a different but related set of treatment strategies into this child's treatment program, and success continued!

Another young child who was almost 2 years old originally appeared to demonstrate very stiff oral-motor movements of the lips, cheeks, tongue, and jaw. I treated the stiffness because she was having difficulty chewing and saying words. This girl improved very well in therapy, and the stiffness began to diminish significantly, but then her oral-motor movements began to appear very floppy! We modified our treatment techniques to meet this new discovery, and her eating and speaking skills continued to improve.

How do these layers develop? In the case of the little girl, she most likely demonstrated floppy movements when she was a baby, but those movements apparently didn't interfere with her ability to breast-feed. Later, as she tried harder and harder to bite, chew, and speak, her movements became stiffer and slower, limiting her ability to function. Thus, by the time I saw her in therapy, the stiffness was masking the underlying floppy movements of the tongue, lips, cheeks, and jaw. I originally felt and saw stiffness but later discovered the underlying floppy movement. We needed to treat the stiffness first. When the floppy movements became apparent, we modified therapy techniques as part of the intervention process.

In hindsight, I discovered a similar situation with the first child I referred to, the little boy whom I initially treated for verbal dyspraxia and later discovered an underlying problem area of mild dysarthria. During further discussion, his mother recalled that he had had some difficulty latching onto the nipple when he was transferring to bottle feeding from breast-feeding. It was not a significant problem, so the medical records hadn't mentioned it. In retrospect, I now realize that the mild dysarthria was the original problem area interfering with latching onto the bottle. Again, as time progressed and this little boy was attempting to learn lots of quick, precise movements of the lips and tongue for sound production, he began demonstrating a significant functional problem in imitating oral movements. Again, the more obvious functional problem area masked the probable initial problem area.

I, as well as a number of other therapists, have treated many children who have progressed along similar paths. Some children have displayed many layers, others a few. In every case, however, new layers did not become evident until we had addressed the initial layers. Based on experience, a therapist often will suspect that another layer could be waiting to be revealed. This is why it is very important to watch for any changes your child might make, and to share your observations with your therapist.

Important Thoughts for Parents

- Ask your therapist to explain and discuss treatment strategies with you.
- Request demonstrations of techniques and therapy strategies that you can incorporate into home activities.
- Discuss with your therapist what movements you should be observing.
- Observe how your child reacts to changes in touch, taste, movement, temperature, lighting, and sounds. Often it's the little changes that yield the biggest discoveries!
- Be certain to inform your therapist about any and all changes you and your family see in your child. Any change is important! As your child's abilities change, therapy techniques should and will change. Your observations are most important. Therapists need your reports.

Problem solving together is exciting, and your child will be the one to benefit!

For more clarification of Neuro-Developmental Treatment (NDT) theory and how it influences therapy for children, see Article 1.2 by Judith Bierman, titled "Philosophy, Theory, and Principles: The What, Why, and How of NDT."

Can I Sign on the Dotted Line??

Regi Boehme, OTR

Over the past 25 years of working with families whose children have special needs, I have observed that parents voice a consistent concern: "Will my child be independent as an adult?" I see three priorities for independence: (a) some form of communication, (b) use of the hands, and (c) some form of mobility.

With our current technology, children can access speech through computers and mobility through electronic chairs and scooters. So even with serious limitations in motor control, children can access communication and mobility.

This article focuses on the development of the signature, an important skill needed for signing checks, filling out application forms, and writing one's name at the end of a computer-written paper or letter. It can make a tremendous difference to the individual who wants to live independently in our society today—the difference between employment and unemployment.

Last night, I was looking at my granddaughter's drawings. Her kindergarten teacher asked everyone in the class to make the same drawing, once a month, from September through June. Each drawing contained three figures—a tree, a house, and a drawing of the child. I spread out all of the monthly drawings in chronological order and saw how much more clearly she was able to express her reality, month by month. There was a big difference between the September and June drawings.

This was the first time I sat with my two granddaughters while their mother and father worked the night shift. We made people out of felt, glue, and paint. We worked with stencils, coloring books, and other crafts. Regardless of which creation they were involved in, each time, the activity was not complete until each printed her name. This was easy for Emily, who was six. But it was not quite as easy for Lydia, who was four. And yet, it was unimportant that some of her letters were backward. What was most important to her was being able to write her name.

Being able to sign one's name is a way to identify one's self as an individual. It brings children a level of pride that we adults take for granted. I learned through living with my husband and son that this personal signature does not need to be legible in order to be legal. But as children grow into adulthood, the signature does require consistency.

Writing involves the ability to hold a pencil or pen. It also involves being able to move the upper arm, lower arm, or wrist. Individuals with motor challenges can create a consistent signature with a very basic grasp and movements of the upper arm alone.

There are many activities that will improve the motor skills used in writing. Finger feeding and self-feeding offer opportunities to explore a variety of grasp patterns. Art work such as finger painting encourages movements of the upper and lower arm and also stimulates movements of the wrist and hand. Finding objects in a container of soapy water, Styrofoam™ chips, noodles, or lentils can stimulate a child's sense of touch. It also encourages movements of the fingers and the whole hand in grasp.

Therapists who use the Neuro-Developmental Treatment (NDT) approach have a knowledge of developmental sequences that can assist them in planning treatment activities. However, they also consider other factors such as task requirements and environmental issues that are critical to motor learning.

Occupational therapists are very creative in making and adapting devices that work for individuals who need them in order to succeed in the same activities as their peers. For example, many products are available that make holding a pencil or pen easier, such as different types of plastic and foam grips. Even children who can't grasp can wear a comfortable splint device that holds the pen for them.

Patience is important. We encourage our children each time we acknowledge their signatures. They feel good about themselves each time we tape their pictures on our refrigerators. Making a scrap book of this art work tells them how valuable their artistic expression is, especially when they have signed on the bottom line!

For more clarification of Neuro-Developmental Treatment (NDT) theory and how it influences therapy for children, see Article 1.2 by Judith Bierman, titled "Philosophy, Theory, and Principles: The What, Why, and How of NDT."

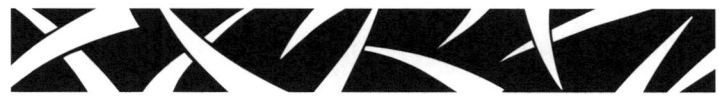

Section 8

Roles

Parents Have Learning Styles Too! How to Help Your Therapist Help You Help Your Child

Marsha Dunn Klein, M.Ed., OTR/L

An important focus of children's therapy programs is on their learning styles—the best ways they can learn. However, children aren't the only ones with a special learning style! What about parents? You, as a parent, have your unique ways of learning and processing information. Therapists will ask you, as a partner in the therapy of your child, to carry over therapy ideas into your home. Do you know your best ways of learning these activities? Have you shared what you know about yourself with your child's therapist? This article will help you discover more about the ways you learn best and how understanding these ways will help you help your child accomplish the everyday home activities that your therapist recommends. What you learn about your own learning needs also can help you better recognize and understand your child's special learning channels. Sharing this critical information with your therapist will help you work more closely together to help your child progress.

A Historic Perspective: Where Did This Home-Program Stuff Come From?

Berta and Karel Bobath, the founders of the Neuro-Developmental Treatment (NDT) approach in London, England, believed that parents need to be a primary component in therapy for young children with cerebral palsy and movement difficulties. They realized that the progress children made in the therapy was dependent on the carryover of therapy ideas into the home. Parents were central to therapeutic progress, and this showed in the Bobaths' teachings.

Prior to the Bobath approach, therapy was considered a series of exercises usually done to the child by the therapist. Home programs, if done at all, often were imitations of specific treatment exercises. Realization that therapy could be translated into everyday home activities was quite a breakthrough in the pediatric therapy field. Through their training courses, the Bobaths helped therapists from around the world understand the importance of taking therapy into the home and incorporating therapeutic techniques into activities of daily living. Therapists began inviting parents into the therapy sessions and demonstrating these home suggestions. As parents became more involved, they shared their ideas with therapists for adapting and refining these therapeutic activities to work in their homes with their own families.

Learning Styles: How We Learn

Educators have long realized that people have different styles of learning. Some are visual learners who need to see something in order to understand it. Others are auditory learners who learn best by listening. Some learn through movement and others through touch. Some learn it once and have it mastered. Others need repetition and reminders. Many folks learn best with a combination of different types of information and different methods of presentation. Therapists and parents traditionally have focused on their children's learning needs. It isn't surprising to realize that we, as adults, have different learning styles, too.

Therefore, if therapists are going to teach parents therapeutic activities, then they must zero-in on the learning style that best matches each parent's learning needs. Therapists can offer these recommendations in a variety of ways to match individual parent learning styles.

You need to figure out your own learning style (unless you are already aware) and make sure you communicate this information to your therapist. See if any of these examples describe you!

- The *Show Me Style*: Many parents want to watch the therapist doing a particular activity and then can imitate it easily. The therapist might demonstrate alternative ways to carry, feed, or present a toy to your child. The *Show Me* method usually works best in person, face to face with the therapist. You can ask questions and discuss strategies.

- The *Read It Style*: Some parents ask to read the information. They seem to learn best from reading the activities on paper. That way they can read more in depth about the theory behind the suggestions and understand the *why*. An advantage of the written word is that you can read it and then look at it again later. Some parents describe fear and confusion at the initial diagnosis of their child. They tell us that getting more information and facts helped them cope and understand.

- The *Tell Me Style*: Some parents ask the therapist to "just tell me" what they should do at home. The therapist might suggest a modification in a bathing routine or a different texture for food. The activity might not need a demonstration—only an explanation.

Your child's therapist can brainstorm with you about different ways to incorporate these ideas into your daily routine.

- The *Let Me Try It Style*: This style often goes hand in hand with the *Show Me* style. To be sure that they fully understand a particular activity, many parents will want the therapist to observe them trying what they understand to be the activity. Many will readily say that "it looks easier than it is!" *Let Me Try It* works for those who need to see, hear, and feel the information in order to really get it. As an example, imagine the therapist demonstrating a special technique to help your child learn to feed him- or herself with a spoon. The therapist suggests that you hold your child's elbow and hand a certain way as you guide scooping and bringing food to the mouth. You can see the demo, hear the explanation, and try it out on your child with the therapist there to give you feedback. You can try it a few times until you are comfortable with it or run out of food to scoop!

- The *Remind Me Style*: This therapy stuff can be overwhelming. *Postural tone this* and *extension that*! Therapists have their own language that could just as easily be Martian! You not only have to get used to the fact that your child needs therapy, but then you also need to learn a whole new language. It's no wonder many parents ask for reminders. Think about what works best for you. Would it help to have a carbon paper take-home sheet for the therapist to write down the suggestions of the day? Or do you like taking your own notes? You can bring your handy-dandy little notebook and jot down what you need. How about a photocopied handout representing that activity in drawings? Perhaps a videotape would help your memory with the fine details, because you can play it over and over with the touch of a button. Some parents like to bring their own video camera to a session to videotape appropriate parts. Other parents bring a tape recorder to tape verbal recommendations, which makes it possible for the parent to listen to the instructions repeatedly until they sink in. An instant photo can be great. Ask the therapist to take a photo of you trying the activity. Put that photo or series of photos in your special-reminder place. You have your own methods of reminders that work for you. Let the therapist know!

- The *Let Me Feel It Style*: For many parents, actually experiencing the therapeutic activity is the most meaningful way for learning and motivation. Many parents tell therapists that they want to feel it themselves, on themselves! Feeling the treatment can help parents know how far to move a leg, how to balance in a certain position, or how the child with a unique set of challenges might feel performing a particular activity of daily living. Many parents have said that they really understood their child better when they tried to imagine what their child feels or experience some of the therapy that their child receives. For some parents, feeling the activity answers the question about why it is necessary. Experiencing the activity can be just what it takes to make the difference.

Lab Experiences

First, try to imagine your body as having the same issues as your child has. Do the home activity the therapist recommends, and feel the problems your child might have with the task. Then think how you need to reorganize that activity so that you can succeed. Chances are that you will have a different level of awareness and a different motivation for helping your child. Here are some examples:

- Close your eyes and try to feed yourself. Notice the challenges that face you. How much of the food did you get in your mouth and how much was on the table or in your lap? What did you have to do to get the food successfully to your mouth? What did you learn that would help you with your child?

- Stiffen your body with your hips bent, your legs out straight and crossed. Tighten your bent elbows at your sides. Fist your hands and bend your wrists down. Shrug your shoulders tight. Now try to balance in the bathtub. How safe do you feel? How independent could you be? How could you pick up and use the soap? What could be done to make you feel safer? Do you need a towel under you so that you slide less? Do you need someone at your side? Imagine what your child is feeling when he or she faces these challenges each day! It makes a difference.

- Imagine yourself, like your child, having a tough time moving one side of your body. Your arm is tight and in a bent position at the elbow. Your whole arm is close to your body. The challenge is to put a shirt on by yourself. Pick a shirt with buttons. Put yourself in the same position as your child. Try putting on the shirt. Discover which strategies work and which don't. Did you notice that the shirt went on more easily when you put your tighter arm in first? What happened when you put it in last? Most parents realize that putting in the tighter arm last is much more difficult because the tightness doesn't allow enough movement to push through the last sleeve hole. By trying to put the shirt on yourself, you can feel the difference in the techniques. Carrying out this home suggestion with your child might be much more meaningful after you have felt what he/she feels and experiences!

- Another way to feel it is to have the therapist do the therapeutic technique on you, moving your ankles through range of motion or actually putting you on the therapy ball to feel the balancing reaction your child experiences. Remember the power of feeling it. Ask the therapist to let you feel the recommendations, or put yourself in your child's shoes (or wheelchair) to understand better the whys and wherefores of therapy.

Did any of these learning styles sound like you? Do you prefer a combination of several? Do you prefer one style for some situations and another style for others? Be aware of what you need. You have your own way of learning. Remember that, your child is in therapy and you're supposed to carry over therapy ideas into your home. Please let the therapist know how to share the information so that it is most meaningful to you. To be most effective, therapy must take place in a strong partnership. Know your learning style so that you can make the most of it!

For more clarification of Neuro-Developmental Treatment (NDT) theory and how it influences therapy for children, see Article 1.2 by Judith Bierman, titled "Philosophy, Theory, and Principles: The What, Why, and How of NDT."

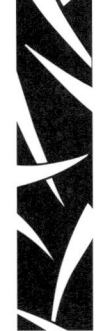

Parents and Therapists as Collaborators in Therapy Programs

8.2

Kristen Birkmeier, M.S., PT

Finding out that your child has a developmental problem can be a very traumatic and scary event for parents. Usually, you receive this information through interactions with a group of professionals who play various roles and who have their own attitudes and biases. By the time you and your child begin to work with a physical, occupational, or speech therapist, you already have met and had your child evaluated by numerous specialists. The information you've already received may have given you hope or dashed your dreams regarding your child and his or her future. You might have had time to come to terms with the information, or you still might be working through this process. Bear in mind that whatever information you have been given regarding your child's future does not necessarily mean that that is what will happen. It is only someone's best effort to give you important facts so that you can process the information and prepare for the future.

This is the time to reach for your brave heart, hold it close, and be sure that you have found a therapist who sees possibilities for your child and his or her future. Finding such a therapist will help you develop important skills that will enable you to take an active role in positively affecting your child's functional ability now and in the future. These parent-therapist relationships usually span over a number of years, and with a little luck, you might have begun a very gratifying parent-professional teaming effort.

Developing a Relationship With Your Therapist

The first time you and your child meet with a therapist is the time to begin developing the collaboration process. The therapist usually is focused on gathering all of the data he or she needs to help set realistic functional goals for your child. These goals are both long term and short term, the time frame being dependent upon the customary practices of the facility in which the therapist works. The therapist should ask you about your concerns and expectations for your child. This is your opportunity to voice any concerns and questions and tell the therapist what dreams and goals you have for your child. If the therapist doesn't ask you, it's important that you make known your concerns, questions, and goals for your child. You should go to this first appointment with the expectation that you and the therapist will work together to develop a therapy program that teaches you the things you need to know and helps your child develop a positive self-image and achieve maximal functional independence.

If you don't come away from an initial interaction with your child's therapist feeling positive and hopeful, or if you're already working with a therapist who doesn't relate to you in this way, perhaps it would be a good idea for you to find another therapist. It isn't important that you develop a friendship with the therapist, but it is very important that you feel respected, listened to, and treated as a partner in your child's therapy program.

Going Through Changes as Your Child Grows Older

As time goes by and you and your child attend regularly scheduled therapy sessions, different phases in your child's growth and development will become important in the treatment program. At these times, it's particularly important for you to voice any concerns or questions you have regarding the plan for your child or different options that might be available. For example, moving from infancy into the toddler phase, from preschooler to the school-age phase, and from preteen to teenager all bring changes that can cause you concern.

Oftentimes, children with cerebral palsy benefit from certain medications and medical treatments or interventions that decrease their muscle tone and delay needed orthopedic surgical procedures for several years. Typically, children need these surgeries between 4 and 6 years of age and again between 10 and 12 years of age. Those are the ages when children go through major growth spurts and their musculature is at greatest risk for getting tight and limiting joint mobility. It is also common for some children to need surgical intervention at these times to lengthen certain muscles or correct bony alignment problems.

It might be helpful for you and your child to meet with a family with an older child who has gone through these treatment options already. It is important that you ask for information and investigate your options so that you can make decisions about your child's care with confidence. Ask your therapist to link you up with another family if you think meeting with them would be helpful.

At other times in your child's growth and development, you might feel overwhelmed with situations you and your child are facing, such as when your toddler turns 3 years old and no longer qualifies for the same services. Many times, this will require that you change therapists or begin taking your child to a facility (or to a different facility) for services rather than having a therapist come to your home. You'll also need to get to know a different service coordinator. It's not unusual for therapists to change from time to time even when you continue with the same program, because therapists usually are a young and very mobile group.

Reaching the age when most children go to kindergarten typically is another difficult time because many children with cerebral palsy don't begin school at the same age as their peers. Any time or age at which most of your friends' children are moving into a new phase or beginning new activities can create stress for your and your child.

When children get to be 7 or 8 years old, they probably will begin to have their own ideas about what they want to work on in therapy. It's important that you make sure your child expresses his or her goals to the therapist in some way, and it's important for you to support these goals. Usually therapists are glad to see this interest develop because it makes therapy goal setting much easier and a lot more fun. Most parents feel that each of these changes is a major event, and each event sometimes causes them concern and emotional upheaval for a time. Open communication with your therapist can help you access new resources and information.

Communicating Well

You'll probably find that the therapist you work with on a regular basis will become a very important person in your life and that of your child. This is especially true if you and your child see the same therapist over a number of years. During this time, many life events will occur in each of your lives, and you probably will share some of the facts about these events with each other, enabling you to get to know each other better. You'll probably find that you are able to talk with your child's therapist about a wide variety of topics and that, over time, a real sense of trust develops. You might find that this sense of trust enables you to seek advice more comfortably and share your fears and concerns. Sometimes you might feel vulnerable, and you'll find that the therapy sessions are a safe place for you to share your concerns and express your feelings.

If, for any reason, you find that you are not comfortable with your child's therapist or with something he or she is doing, you owe it to the therapist to discuss your concerns. Conflict usually arises when the two parties don't discuss a misunderstanding or difference of opinion. The conflict goes unresolved until one of you is able to bring up the issue for discussion. The ability to listen becomes particularly important in conflict resolution. Usually, you'll be able to resolve the misunderstanding through honest and open communication with each other. Doing this in person is best, but telephone contact can be just as effective if face-to-face contact is not possible.

Collaboration requires ongoing and open communication between you and your child's therapist. You both have something very important to contribute when you work together to help your child achieve his or her true physical potential. Finding out that your child has a developmental problem certainly can be a very traumatic and scary event for parents. Teaming with a therapist who has your best interests, as well as your child's, at heart is the best way to enable you to take an active role in positively affecting your child's functional ability now and in the future.

For more clarification of Neuro-Developmental Treatment (NDT) theory and how it influences therapy for children, see Article 1.2 by Judith Bierman, titled "Philosophy, Theory, and Principles: The What, Why, and How of NDT."

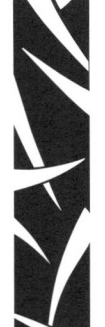

Divide Up the Tasks, Not the Body Parts

Marybeth Trapani-Hanasewych, M.S., CCC-SLP

Who's in Charge?

As a parent, you are the only one who sees every part of your child's life. Clinicians, therapists, teachers, and other child-care workers see only one time frame in your child's day.

Therapists and families can become so involved in each of the specialty areas of speech and language, gross-or fine motor-activities, or cognitive skills that they begin to think that a speech-language pathologist works only with talking and eating, an occupational therapist works with the hands, a physical therapist works with walking, and the teacher works on cognitive (thinking) skills. The problem with that kind of process is that the child gets very divided as he/she gives attention to each task, working in pieces instead of as a whole unit.

But you, the parent, are the captain of the ship, the only person able to help pull the child's entire program and life together. You are the boss.

The Neuro-Developmental Treatment (NDT) philosophy states:

> NDT is a problem-solving approach that involves the treatment and management of individuals with movement dysfunction. The person is addressed as a whole and therefore the process is individualized and includes an interdisciplinary team.

Functional Example

An example of the decision-making process involving the whole child and the entire team is the decision to introduce switches. If your child is now using or might use a switch for play or a communication system, the team must consider the whole child in making the decision. Each member of the team has equal importance in the decision. Remember that some members of the team might be more experienced than others. As a parent, you must make the decision as a member of your child's team.

Criteria for Decision Making

The following example describes how all team members contribute to the decision-making process

Child: The child enjoys watching a battery-operated toy run or likes to use a BIGmack™ switch—an augmentative device—to give directions or make a verbal request. (The BIGmack switch is a simple communication system that has two features. It can record a single message that's 10–20 seconds long. It is much like a tape recorder except that it records only short messages. When the child activates the switch, the message replays. The second feature allows a battery-operated toy to be connected to the switch and turned on when the child activates the switch.)

Parent: The parent wants to help the child to enjoy life, have fun, and be able to communicate. As parents, we want it all for our children. Our financial resources always are a concern in deciding what we want or can afford for our children. We need the resources to be functional and reliable as well.

Speech-Language Pathologist: This therapist might look at the following parameters:

a. What are your child's cognitive skills and how will a simple switch or a BIGmack switch help improve them?

b. How can the equipment be used now to prepare also for the future? For example, rather than using a single-switch toy that requires the child to hit and hold the switch in order to keep the toy activated, try to encourage the use of a latch timer. It allows the switch to work the toy as a toggle (on/off) or for a few seconds (as a timer), after which the child will need to hit the switch to reactivate the toy. Why? There is no augmentative speech communication device that works on a hit-and-hold pattern. All the devices require a hit-and-release pattern. A latch timer will begin to prepare the child to use other augmentative systems or access a computer.

c. A BIGmack can be used so in many different ways. Here are a few examples:

Recorded Message	Possible Use
"I want more, please."	The child uses the switch to play a message requesting more bubbles or food.
Connect the switch to the battery-operated toy.	The child makes the request and the toy activates.
"Turn the page."	While reading a book together, the adult waits the child to use the switch before turning the next page.
"I want a kiss."	The recipient of the request gives the child a kiss after the message is played.

Occupational Therapist: The OT might be looking at the fine-motor skills needed to access the switch. Which is the best position? Can the child use it during floor play, at the kitchen table, or on a parent's lap?

Physical Therapist: Physical therapy might focus on communicating in standing or during gait training (walking). How can a switch work during these times? Parents and professionals need to share information about which devices are available and then problem solve about how to use these devices.

Teacher: How can teachers use switches in the classroom in a functional manner? A classroom job such as line leader works well with a switch. The child could request "Follow me" using the switch and then lead the line of children to another class.

All other important folks in a child's life (grandparents, neighbors, friends, bus drivers, or aides): Some of the best ideas come from these folks. The challenge for the team is to gather input from all these people.

Communication

Professionals are responsible for communicating with one another. However, connecting with one another can be difficult and very time consuming. The ideas listed here suggest how a parent might help to facilitate that communication in order to divide up the tasks and not the body parts.

1. Use a communication logbook. This can be any kind of notebook. If your child helps to decorate the book, it then becomes part of the child's property and he or she is more emotionally invested in it. All therapists, teachers, parents, grandparents, aides, and anyone who comes in contact with the child can use the book to communicate with anyone else who interacts with that child. It works best when the parents gently remind the therapists to make an entry. The book then acts as a log of progress for later review.

2. Make sure you, the parent, have access to all the information. However, remember that you are not responsible for communication between professionals.

3. Insist on communication at those critical decision points throughout your child's life. Remember that you and the child are the consumers and can request a family conference.

These are only a few suggestions. A combination of these suggestions usually works best. It depends on everyone to ensure that the tasks are divided up, not the body parts.

For more clarification of Neuro-Developmental Treatment (NDT) theory and how it influences therapy for children, see Article 1.2 by Judith Bierman, titled "Philosophy, Theory, and Principles: The What, Why, and How of NDT."

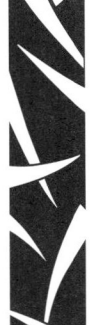

Team Goals and Roles: How Parents Can Assure Continuity of Care

Diane Berg McCormack, M.S., OTR

Every family deals with stress and learns to cope with the demands of caring for a new baby. However, families who have a child with disabilities also must struggle with new information and issues that invade their daily lives. Parents who still might be in the process of grieving for the loss of an expected healthy child must adapt to the demands of their child's disability. Additional therapy-related caregiving tasks can cause strains on the family that jeopardize the child's overall needs.

If therapy services are so limited that the child has few opportunities to practice new skills, parents might need to access additional resources. Home health aides or nurses can assist with therapy and nursing care. Unfortunately, along with the need for these services comes the dilemma for parents and therapists of continually having to train home-health aides and nurses because of high turnover rates. When so many people are working with the child, especially over time, maintaining communication and continuity of care is difficult. Parents can facilitate this process by being very clear with other team members about the needs of their child and family. As a part of the team, the family's contributions can assure continuity of care and enhance progress toward the child's functional goals.

This article outlines the process necessary for creating an effective team program. The example that follows outlines the goal of increasing the child's ability to function in standing throughout the day.

Needs and Goals

What are the specific impairments (e.g., poor shoulder-girdle control, tight hamstrings, or poor breath support) that relate both to therapy needs (e.g., weight bearing and shifting, elongation of musculature, or rib cage-expansion) and to daily life (e.g., standing upright during self-care activities)? How can your family and the rest of the team best address these needs and set objectives for activities throughout the day; that is, at home with the family and/or home-health staff and at school?

The first step in the team process is to summarize the tasks and related goals that will enable your child to participate in daily activities. For example, if a primary need of your child is to stand for longer periods during the day, each team member might address this goal with a different emphasis by using a different variety of activities while the child is in supported standing.

Family

As a family member, your child needs to increase his or her social experiences and self-concept. Standing provides a different perception of the environment. It means being tall enough to interact with other family members in an upright position. It can increase the child's ability to be a functional family member. For example, when upright, your child can wash or dry dishes more efficiently because he can see inside the sink and the tops of the kitchen counters. Participating in family chores encourages the development of prevocational or work skills needed to be a productive member of society.

Physical therapy

The physical therapist might want to increase your child's ability to stand upright with support so that she can expand her exploration of the environment and increase her ability to transfer independently.

Occupational therapy

The occupational therapist might view upright standing as a great position for increasing your child's hand skills, manipulating objects that assist with activities of daily living.

Speech therapy

The speech-language pathologist might want to increase your child's ability to initiate and maintain a conversation, which might be easier when standing upright due to head and trunk alignment that facilitates eye contact, respiratory support, and coordination of posture while vocalizing and communicating needs.

Roles

What are the tasks that best match the roles of the family, the therapist, the home-health caregiver, and the school? Each team member (parent, therapist, educator, nurse, and aide) is a unique individual with experience or training in specific areas of care. The second step in the team process helps answer these questions by reviewing the child's daily schedule and determining how each member can address the child's goals most effectively. Parents can sew a thread of continuity throughout their child's day, in and out of the home and with a variety of caregivers, in order to increase the child's ability to tolerate the upright posture.

Table 1: Impairments, Therapy Needs, and Examples of Functional Tasks: An NDT Perspective for Standing in a Stander

Impairment	Therapy Needs	Functional Tasks
Social (Family)	Social difficulties (dependent in many tasks)	Participation as a productive family member; standing upright independently in a stander
		Folding towels while in the stander, as a family chore or for extra money
Motor (Physical Therapy)	Muscle stiffness in hamstrings and heel cords	Neuromuscular inhibition techniques to modulate tone prior to standing; prolonged weight bearing to stretch shortened muscles
		Watching birds come to a window bird feeder
	Muscle weakness in neck and trunk muscles (especially flexors)	Proper head and trunk support systems and practicing motor skills in a semireclined (but upright) position for muscle alignment and strengthening
		Batting at a balloon attached to the ceiling (tray removed)
Motor (Occupational Therapy)	Poor muscle coactivation of head and shoulder girdle	Weight bearing and shifting movements of elbows on a tray attached to the stander
		Rocking on elbows to music on a radio or music video
	Overuse of immature movement patterns in arms and hands	Proper positioning in upright with tray support to facilitate more mature and functional arm and hand movements
		Multisensory fine-motor experiences such as rolling cookie dough, buttering toast, or stirring pudding
	Sensory processing difficulties	Utilization of sensory diet strategies when upright to facilitate functional tasks
		Playing at a water or sand table
Speech and Language (Speech Therapy)	Limited initiation of conversation	Role models to facilitate active participation of conversation
		Playing games that require verbalization with a peer or adult in standing
	Inability to sustain speech	Neuromuscular facilitation techniques to modulate muscle coactivation and coordination of movements of the rib cage prior to standing
		Singing into a karaoke microphone with a peer while standing

Family's role

Ask your child's therapists to teach all family members proper positioning of your child in a standing frame and the proper way to transfer your child in and out of adaptive equipment such as a wheelchair or gait trainer. If the child is going to use a static (stationary) stander, focus on ways to include the child in daily home routines, such as:

- standing at a counter or sink in the kitchen and assisting with meal or baking preparations
- standing at a table to work on a project or play a game
- positioned at the living room window to look outdoors and observe the weather and neighborhood activities

Home-health-care staff's role

Nurses (RNs and LPNs) and home-health aides can receive training for proper placement in static positioning devices and ways to transfer your child safely in and out of equipment such as the stander, which could become a part of the daily routines for brushing teeth, combing hair, and playing.

Teacher's and teacher's aide's role

Teachers and aides also can learn proper positioning of your child in a stander, as well as ways to transfer the child in and out of other equipment. The stander would become a part of your child's educational day for working on learning activities.

Therapist's role

In a school setting, physical, occupational, and speech therapists will consider handling, positioning, and adaptive equipment needs as they relate to education, provided by direct or indirect services. The therapists address activities involving a standing frame, gait trainer, or standing with external support, in terms of how such activities relate to function during the school day.

Physical, occupational, and speech therapists might have different treatment emphases depending on their training, work situations, and theoretical philosophies. As parents get to know their child's therapists, they can ask about each therapist's background and request explanations of terminology and treatment emphasis. This knowledge-sharing assists the communication process and enhances continuity of care.

Traditional or eclectic physical therapists might emphasize the components needed for standing and mobility during functional tasks throughout the day. Traditional occupational therapists might address the use of upper extremities for daily living skills, visual perceptual tasks, and self-care activities while in the upright position. Traditional speech therapists might address oral motor function and respiratory/phonatory abilities in the upright posture, relating them to daily speech and language activities. These services can be direct or indirect, depending on the service provider's program.

Physical, occupational, and speech therapists with Neuro-Developmental Treatment (NDT) training also will address traditional therapy needs for standing abilities with a more dynamic handling and positioning emphasis during direct hands-on therapy. See Table 1, Impairments, Therapy Needs, and Examples of Functional Tasks: An NDT Perspective for Standing in a Stander.

Continuity of Care

How can you and your family work together with the rest of the multiagency team to provide continuity of care in a variety of environments?

As parents, you can help define the roles for each team member in either a formal or informal manner. Even if children receive services from home-care nursing or aides, they typically spend most of their time with their families. Children spend the next largest amount of time with school staff or home-health caregivers and the least amount of time in direct therapy. However, therapists can facilitate therapeutic handling and positioning throughout the child's entire day by teaching and training families and other team members.

Parents and therapists working with home-care staff sometimes find that constant turnover of nurses or aides makes it very difficult to train these individuals for proper handling, positioning, transfers, and monitoring of range of motion. Videotaping inservice training gives agencies the flexibility to train staff as needed. Tape instant photos of proper positioning and handling techniques to a wall in your home to assist in caregiver training, and send copies of these photos to school as a quick guide for the classroom teacher and aide.

Summary

Continuity of care for your child with a disability requires that you be willing to communicate and share important information with your team. By addressing your child's impairments, needs, and goals, and defining family and caregiver roles, you can help your child achieve functional skills for participating as fully as possible in daily living activities in the home, school, and community environments.

For more clarification of Neuro-Developmental Treatment (NDT) theory and how it influences therapy for children, see Article 1.2 by Judith Bierman, titled "Philosophy, Theory, and Principles: The What, Why, and How of NDT."

What Does My Child Need and How Can I Help? Application and Philosophy of NDT According to the Bobaths

Joan Mohr, PT

If parents and therapists were to consider what factors contribute to a successful therapy program, they probably would agree that communication among team members should be at the top of the list.

What do therapists need to learn from you, the parents? What do you need to learn from them? And most important, what do parents and therapists need to learn from the child?

As the therapists evaluate your child, they need to learn from you. They need to know how you see the child's needs and difficulties, what information you've received from your physicians, and why your child has been sent to therapy. In addition, they need you to tell them what your own needs are as you interact with your child. It's important to hear from both parents because moms and dads are different. They have different views, opinions, and needs. If there are other children in the family, therapists also must consider their questions about their brother or sister with special needs.

Your therapists should share their observations and findings with you by describing everything your child is able to do. They then should explain what they think the reasons are for your child not being able to accomplish certain tasks that other children of similar age can do.

During the therapists' explanations, it is your responsibility as parents to stop them at any time if you don't understand completely, and to ask questions or request more detail and clarification. Often, questions will come up in your mind at a later time when you're not with the therapist. Many parents have discovered that it's a good idea to write down comments and questions on a small note pad so that they will be sure to remember them during their next visit. These written questions are especially helpful when only one parent is able to come to the therapy session and the other parent has questions, too. The notepad is one tool to help keep communication open. It also can provide a way for parents to keep a record of the therapist's comments and instructions.

Remember that although therapists can help you with many questions, it is physicians who provide a diagnosis or prognosis. Therapists can offer an opinion, based upon their experience, about your child's progress, but it is even more important for you to tell the therapists your opinion and to relay any frustrations you might feel because you hoped for and expected more. Experienced therapists then might be able to help give you perspective by discussing examples of their experiences with other children.

From the very beginning of the Neuro-Developmental Treatment (NDT) approach, which was developed in the early 1940s by Berta and Karel Bobath, parents of children with disabilities always were included as major members of the team. Back then, this was a novel concept. As a parent, you should be involved and receive information on all aspects of your child's therapies so that you can make informed, appropriate decisions. The therapists' job is to supply the information to help you make the decision, but it is you who are ultimately responsible for your child. In other words, the professionals are there to help but not to decide for you. They might have suggestions, but they must try to be objective and help you see all sides of each issue.

The role that you play in handling your child at home is extremely important. The Bobaths always said that what the therapist does in treatment needs to be carried out in daily life. This means that therapists should show you how to prepare and assist your child in different functions during the day. This should not be a long list of exercises but rather a few purposeful activities that the child needs to learn in order to achieve the best quality of function.

Since moms and dads each relate differently to their child, therapists need to help each parent participate in the activities that best complement the expression of those differences. You can help your therapists understand not only the individual parent/child relationships that exist in your family but also the effects of the specific dynamics in your child's background and home environment. Only in this way will therapists be able to relate to your child and other family members appropriately. For example, in some cultures the mother has total responsibility for the child's upbringing until a certain age, when the responsibility shifts to the father. In other cultures, the father, not the mother, is the main person who will assume the role of assisting in therapy-related activities. In addition, grandparents, especially grandmothers, have significant roles in many cultures as authoritarian figures and/or caregivers.

As you receive various home programs, your therapists have the responsibility to make the programs realistic and suited to your abilities and home situations. This requires your help and honest input. It is your responsibility as parents to tell a therapist if you are having difficulty carrying out the home program. This might be due to the

What Does My Child Need and How Can I Help? Application and Philosophy of NDT According to the Bobaths

requirements of physical handling, your child's overwhelming medical problems, or too many other household and family responsibilities. Therapists periodically should ask you to demonstrate exactly what you are doing at home to make sure that you have been given proper instructions and that the program is working for you in your particular circumstances. The therapist then might modify the activities, encouraging those activities needed to help the child perform a task while avoiding those that might not be helpful. Therapists also should review basic principles every once in awhile to reinforce and ensure mutual understanding between the therapist and the parents.

This concept of handling skills as performed by you and family members has been geared toward helping the child with a disability develop into an active member of the family, community, and society. Although the carryover into the home by you, the parents and family, can be a difficult task, it can become easier when therapists use therapy time to teach hands-on techniques to you so that you will become more confident as you practice the techniques over and over in your home.

Your therapist will guide your hands so that you experience the correct movements and provide the best quality of movement possible to gain the maximum control and development of muscles and joints. Your goal is for your child to take over more and more control of the movement until it is possible to complete the task independently. The best quality of movement is important. Poor movement patterns, if left uncorrected, develop into further restriction of movement in the future, which may lead to problems with painful, stiff muscles and joints. Even with the best handling possible provided by the therapist and carried over and sustained by you, these problems aren't always eliminated, but most certainly they will be kept to a minimum.

Communication is the key. You must let your therapists know your feelings about your ability to carry over what you have been taught, exactly which tasks you feel you are able to carry out, and which ones are difficult or impossible. Be sure to share your feelings about time constraints and other pressures.

What can parents do to help their children become more active participants in family and community life? As they assist their children to participate physically as much as possible in different tasks, parents' hands will need to be guiding their children's actions to achieve success with the best quality of movement. If the children's disability doesn't allow much functional movement, they still can participate by directing the activity. For example, during dressing, they not only can push their arms into the sleeves or legs into the pants but, if appropriate, they also can decide which shirt or outfit they wish to wear. Another example might be to encourage children to invite certain friends to come and play, and to choose which games they would like to play. Parents also can ask their children to direct the way to the market, to help choose the food to buy, and to indicate on which shelf a food item is located. If their children aren't able to perform these types of skills well or at all, the therapist needs to know, so that he/she can incorporate these skills into the therapy plan as a functional task. All of these activities will help children initiate action and interaction, instead of remaining passive and dependent.

Children with disabilities need to learn responsibility for their actions and the difference between right and wrong. In terms of discipline, parents need to maintain boundaries and help their children learn to distinguish between appropriate and inappropriate behavior, just as other children do. All this is part of developing character as well as life skills, which they will need in the future. Children also need times and opportunities to play independently, so that they can enjoy doing things by themselves and are not always dependent on others.

Although children with disabilities need extra time and special attention, parents also need to make time for other family members and for themselves.

This article emphasizes the importance of you and your child as team members. Teamwork depends on open, honest communication. You need to understand all aspects of your child's needs so that you can make appropriate, informed decisions. This responsibility always should be in your hands.

For more clarification of Neuro-Developmental Treatment (NDT) theory and how it influences therapy for children, see Article 1.2 by Judith Bierman, titled "Philosophy, Theory, and Principles: The What, Why, and How of NDT."

References for Parents

Adams, R. C., Daniel, A. H., & Rullman, L. (1982). *Games, sports, and exercises for the physically handicapped* (3rd ed.). Philadelphia: Lea & Febiger.

Allbright, A. L. (1997, September). Current treatments for spasticity: An informed partnership—Family and pediatrician. *Exceptional Parent Magazine*, 73–77.

Batshaw, M. L. (1997). *Children with disabilities* (4th ed.). Baltimore: Paul H. Brookes.

Brinson, C. L. (Ed.). (1982). *The helping hand: A manual describing methods for handling the young child with cerebral palsy*. Charlottesville, VA: Children's Rehabilitation Center, University of Virginia.

Cross, M. (1987). *Wait for me!* New York: Random House in conjunction with the Children's Television Workshop.

Diamond, S. (1981). Growing up with parnets of a handicapped child: A handicapped person's perspective. In J. L. Paul (Ed.), *Understanding and working with parents of children with special needs*, (pp.23–50). New York: Holt, Reinhart & Winston.

Dickman, I., & Gordon, S. (1985). *One miracle at a time: How to get help for your disabled child—From the experience of other parents*. New York: Simon & Schuster.

Erhardt, R. P. (1991-1992, Winter). Improving visual control: Activities for parents and infants. *Team Talk, 1*, 12–15 (available from Team Talk, P.O. Box 83165, Milwaukee, WI 53223).

Exley, H. (1984). *What it's like to be me* (2nd ed.). New York: Friendship Press.

Fassler, J. (1975). *Howie helps himself*. Niles, IL: Albert Whitman.

Featherstone, H. (1982). *A difference in the family: Life with a disabled child*. New York: Penguin.

Finnie, N. (1997). *Handling the young cerebral palsy child at home* (3rd ed.). New York: E. P. Dutton.

Fraser, B. A., & Hensinger, R. N. (1983). *Managing physical handicaps: A practical guide for parents, care providers, and educators*. Baltimore: Paul H. Brookes.

Friedberg, J. B., Mullins, J. B., & Sukiennik, A. W. (1985). *Accept me as I am: Best books of juvenile nonfiction on impairments and disabilities*. New York: R. R. Bowker.

Geralis, E. (Ed.). (1998). *Children with cerebral palsy: A parents' guide* (2nd ed.). Rockville, MD: Woodbine House.

Good, J. D., & Reis, J. G. (1985). *A special kind of parenting: Meeting the needs of handicapped children*. Franklin Park, IL: La Leche League International.

Harrison, H., & Kositsky, A. (1981). *The premature baby book*. New York: St. Martin's Press.

Jaeger, L., & Gertz, J. (1997). *Home program instruction sheets for infants and children* (4th ed.). San Antonio, TX: Therapy Skill Builders.

Jones, M. L. (1980). *Home care for the chronically ill or disabled child*. New York: Harper & Row.

Klein, M. D., & Delaney, T. A. (1994). *Feeding and nutrition for the child with special needs. Handouts for parents*. San Antonio, TX: Therapy Skill Builders.

Koomar, J., & Friedman, B. (1998). *The hidden senses: Your balance sense*. Hugo, MN: PDP.

Koomar, J., & Friedman, B. (1998). *The hidden senses: Your muscle sense*. Hugo, MN: PDP.

Kriegsman, K. H., Zaslow, E. L., & D'Mura-Rechsteiner, J. (1992). *Taking charge: Teenagers talk about life and physical disabilities*. Rockville, MD: Woodbine House.

Lindemann, J. E., & Lindemann, S. J. (1988). *Growing up proud: A parents' guide to the psychological care of children with disabilities*. New York: Warner Books.

Meyer, D. (Ed.). (1995). *Uncommon fathers: Reflections on raising a child with a disability*. Rockville, MD: Woodbine House.

Meyer, D. J., Vadasy, P. F., & Fewell, R. R. (1996). *Living with a brother or sister with special needs* (2d ed.). Seattle, WA: University of Washington Press.

Miller, F., Bachrach, S. J., Boos, M. L., Duffy, L., & Pearson, D. T. (1997). *Cerebral palsy: A complete guide for caregiving*. Baltimore: Johns Hopkins University.

Miller, N. B. (1994). *Nobody's perfect—Living and growing with children who have special needs*. Baltimore: Paul H. Brooks.

Mollan, R. (1981). *Yes they can! A handbook for effectively parenting the handicapped*. Buena Park, CA: Reality Productions.

Moore, C. (1990). *A reader's guide for parents of children with mental, physical, or emotional disabilities*. Rockville, MD: Woodbine House.

References

Morris, L. R., & Schulz, L. (1989). *Creative play activities for children with disabilities: A resource book for teachers and parents* (2nd ed.). Champaign, IL: Human Kinetics.

Murphy, J. (1982). *Home care of handicapped children: A guide.* Lyons, CO: Carol L. Lutey.

Musselwhite, C. R. (1987). *Adaptive play for special needs children: Strategies to enhance communication and learning.* Boston: College-Hill.

Perske, R., Clifton, A., McClean, B. M., & Stein, J. I. (Eds.). (1986). *Mealtimes for persons with severe handicaps.* Baltimore: Paul H. Brookes.

Piper, W. (1954). *The little engine that could.* New York: Platt & Munk.

Powell, T., & Ogle, P. (1993). *Brothers and sisters: A special part of exceptional families* (2nd ed.). Baltimore: Paul H. Brookes.

Pueschel, S. M., Scala, P. S., Weidenman, L. E., & Bernier, J. C. (Eds.). (1995). *The special child: A source book for parents of children with developmental disabilities* (2nd ed.). Baltimore: Paul H. Brookes.

Russell, P. (1985). *The wheelchair child: How handicapped children can enjoy life to its fullest* New York: Prentice Hall.

Sadler, M. (1983). *It's not easy being a bunny.* New York: Random House.

Schleichkorn, J. (1983). *Coping with cerebral palsy: Answers to questions parents often ask.* Austin, TX: Pro-Ed.

Schleifer, M. J., & Klein, S. G. (Eds.). (1985). *The disabled child and the family: An exceptional parent reader.* Boston: The Exceptional Parent.

Schwartz, S., & Miller, J. E. H. (1988). *The language of toys: Teaching communication skills to special-needs children.* Rockville, MD: Woodbine House.

Scott, E. P., Jan, J. E., & Freeman, R. D. (1995). *Can't your child see?* (3rd ed.). Austin, TX: Pro-Ed.

Southall, I. (1968). *Let the balloon go.* New York: Bradbury Press.

Stein, S. B. (1974). *About handicaps: An open family book of parents and children together.* New York: Walker.

Thompson, C. E. (1986). *Raising a handicapped child: A helpful guide for parents of the physical disabled.* New York: William Morrow.

Whinston, J. L. (1989). *I'm Joshua and "Yes I can."* New York: Vantage.